OSTEOPATHY

ALTERNATIVE HEALTH

OSTEOPATHY

STEPHEN SANDLER

ILLUSTRATED BY SHAUN WILLIAMS

An OPTIMA book

© Stephen Sandler 1987

First published in 1987 by
Macdonald Optima, a division of
Macdonald & Co. (Publishers) Ltd

A BPCC PLC company

British Library Cataloguing in Publication Data

Sandler, Stephen
    Osteopathy.—(Alternative health)
    1. Osteopathy
    I. Title
    615.5′33   RZ341

    ISBN 0-356-12428-2

Macdonald & Co. (Publishers) Ltd
3rd Floor
Greater London House
Hampstead Road
London NW1 7QX

Printed and bound in Great Britain by
Hazell Watson & Viney Ltd
Member of the BPCC Group
Aylesbury
Bucks

CONTENTS

1.
WHAT IS OSTEOPATHY?

Osteopathy is a system of diagnosis and treatment that lays its main emphasis on the structural and mechanical problems of the body. It is concerned with the body's framework and how it functions, because osteopathy is based on the theory that the musculoskeletal system is more than just a scaffolding from which the body's organs hang. Osteopathy is not a universal panacea for all ills and does not claim to be. Rather, it is a unique system of both diagnosis and treatment that can be immensely helpful to people with problems that originate or are reflected in the musculoskeletal system of the body.

Osteopaths are concerned with total body health. They believe that the body's skeletal structures and organ systems are of equal importance to normal health and that the relationship between the two is mutually interdependent. So, by examining and understanding the functions of the body's organic systems and exploring the interrelationship between these systems and the musculoskeletal system, osteopaths believe they can guide patients towards better health and therefore less disease.

Osteopaths are practitioners of manual medicine; in other words, they work with their hands both to diagnose conditions and to treat them. Osteopaths use palpation, feeling the tissues under their fingers, and by comparing the temperature, tone, shape and response to movement to what they know to be normal, decide how best manually to treat the patient.

THE BEGINNINGS OF OSTEOPATHY

Osteopathy was founded in America in 1874 by Dr Andrew Taylor Still of Kirksville, Missouri. Dr Still was a doctor in a small frontier town in the mid-West. Life for a country doctor in those days was very different from what it is today. There were no pain-killing drugs, X-rays or other hospital tests. The local apothecary or chemist, if there was one, sold little more than remedies based on herbs and folklore, for modern pharmacology was as much in its infancy as medicine. The germ theory of disease put forward by Lister and Pasteur was still unheard of, so even if patients undergoing surgery survived the terrible

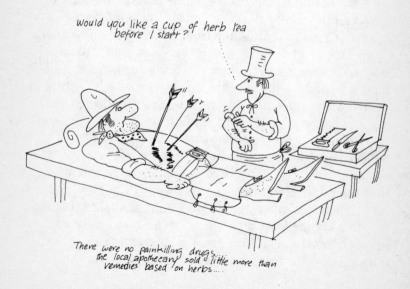

Would you like a cup of herb tea before I start?

There were no painkilling drugs, the local apothecary sold little more than remedies based on herbs....

ordeal of an operation without anaesthetic, they often died from an infection soon afterwards.

Medical training was in no better state. There were few medical schools and those that existed were very expensive, so there was little opportunity for anyone wishing to enter the medical profession. Dr Still was fortunate. As the son of a doctor he went to medical school and received a formal training. After finishing this, he worked with his father. Doing the rounds of his rural practice he particularly noticed the way his patients' health was affected by the way they used their bodies.

STRUCTURE GOVERNS FUNCTION

Early in his career, Dr Still realized one of the basic principles of osteopathy, which is as true today as it was then: structure governs function. In other words, if the body is correctly adjusted there will be minimal stress and tension to the supporting tissues of muscles and joints, and so the body is likely to function correctly. Following on from this, he maintained that, given the right circumstances, the body has the power to heal itself.

As an analogy, think of how a mechanic works on a car. If, for example, the tyres are wearing unevenly, you would not only expect the mechanic to change them but also to examine the vehicle to find out why the tyres are wearing unevenly. So it is with osteopathy and musculoskeletal-based pain. The osteopath is concerned quite as much with the reasons *why* a problem occurs as with the problem itself. It matters not if the problem is acute or chronic, a few hours or a few weeks old; it is the reasons behind the breakdown in function that are important to an osteopathic diagnosis.

A good example of this is a common problem many osteopaths are asked to treat. An athlete suffers an injury while out running. The medical history alone might reveal a tear in the thigh or hamstring muscles. On careful examination, however, the osteopath might find that there is also evidence of a previous injury at the level of the ankle or lower back which has led to the formation of inelastic scar tissue. This now means that the thigh muscles are being asked not only to develop according to the demands placed upon them by the athlete's training programme, but also to accommodate scar tissue in other places caused by the previous injury. Without attention to the old scar tissue as well as to the new injury, the athlete will soon break down again.

This example also illustrates why, on your first visit (see Chapter 4) you will be asked for a detailed medical history and examined in areas of the body which do not hurt and are not close to the part that does.

In dealing with chronic pain, for example chronic low back ache, osteopaths do not believe that it is enough to treat patients with drugs that mask the pain or reduce the inflammation in the muscles. Instead, they look at the causes and predispositions in that patient's lifestyle in an attempt not only to treat the acute manifestation of the pain but to prevent it from recurring once it has been treated. And this type of 'treatment' may take the form of practical suggestions, such as getting yourself a better and more supportive chair if you have a sedentary job (see Chapter 6 for more suggestions).

2.
BACKS, DISCS AND OSTEOPATHS

Back pain brings more patients to an osteopath's consulting rooms than any other problem. In fact back pain and the related syndromes of sciatica, lumbago or the so-called trapped nerve, account for about 75 per cent of an osteopath's work.

After coughs, colds and emotionally related disorders, low back pain of one type or another is the fourth most common problem that GPs are asked to treat. In any day in Britain more than 100,000 people will be away from work with low back pain and its related disorders. 100,000 people represents Wembley football stadium filled to capacity on Cup Final day or 2,000 double-decker buses full of passengers. And these illustrations, of course, only represent the people who are away from work — there are literally millions more who somehow manage to stay at work despite their pain. In financial terms this represents millions of pounds of lost time and production in industry each year.

Most major problems have many causes and some that

have not yet even been discovered. Low back pain is no exception. Below are some of the reasons why so many of us suffer as we do from our backs.

THE UPRIGHT POSTURE

Ancient skeletons recovered from archeological sites show that humans have probably suffered from back pain ever since they first made the transition from walking on all fours to walking upright. The vertebrae in these ancient skeletons show the tell-tales signs of wear and tear and degenerative change that must in some cases have been very painful indeed.

Humans do not have the structural advantage of spreading their weight over all four limbs as do most other mammals. Instead our weight is carried via the spine, the pelvis and the discs, those troublesome pads of shock absorbing gristle that separate the vertebrae of our backs. Four-legged animals have a low body mass with front and

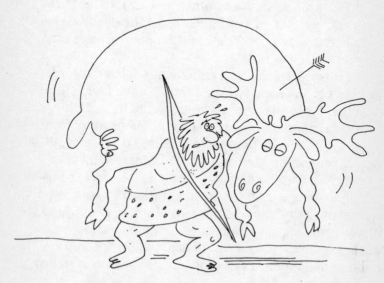

The vertebrae in ancient skeletons show signs of wear and tear...

back supports, whereas a human's body mass is higher and carried vertically. Four-legged animals need little effort to maintain balance, whereas we need a complicated set of muscles both in front and behind our centre of gravity just to stop us falling over.

It wouldn't be so bad if humans carried their weight in one piece, but they don't. There are seven cervical vertebrae, twelve thoracic vertebrae, and five lumbar vertebrae all balanced like a pile of bricks on the solid bony pelvis. When we walk, stand, sit and so on, each action has to be coordinated and held carefully in balance, otherwise even the simplest of movements will soon become impossible.

THE SPINAL CURVES

Front and back curves

Our spines are not straight lines. If you look at someone from the side, you can see a number of different curves that are either concave to the front or concave to the back. These are known as kyphoses and lordoses respectively.

Babies begin to develop muscles at the backs of their necks from the moment they are put on their stomachs and start lifting their heads. These muscles grow thicker and stronger the more they are used. They will help to pull the head back and the chin up and soon the babies will develop their normal cervical lordoses.

Likewise when a child starts to crawl, the tummy will hang down pulling the spine along with it. So the lumbar lordosis in the small of the back develops.

The contents of the chest cavity and the angles of the ribs will develop the dorsal kyphosis, and the sacrum or flat bone at the base of the spine will come to lie at a slight angle to the pelvic bones and so the final sacral kyphosis is formed.

In other words, normal development gives four evenly balanced curves in the anterior/posterior plane — two lordoses and two kyphoses. Unfortunately, however,

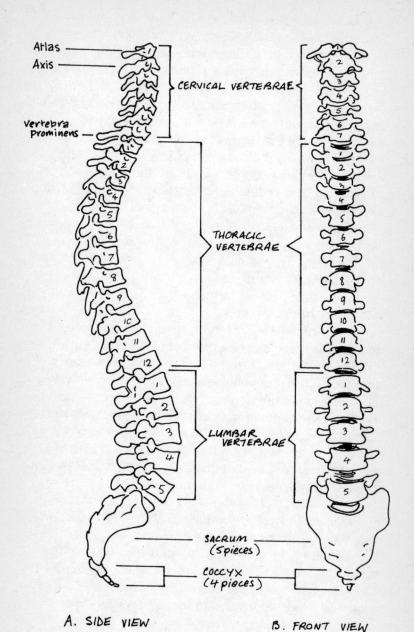

THE VERTEBRAL COLUMN

various factors can and do occur which may cause these front to back curves to flatten or deepen, leading to the appearance of round shoulders or a sagging pot belly. In the lumbar region of the spine (see diagram on page 16) it can cause an exaggerated folding of the ligaments or shortening of the muscles. Young girls with larger busts than their friends often try to hide the fact by pulling their shoulders forward, so causing the dorsal spine to become round. There is also a condition known as osteochondrosis, which is very common indeed in the spine, causing a flattening or stiffening that affects the spinal ligaments and wedges together groups of vertebrae.

From this it is obvious that the normal development of these front to back curves will give normal spinal function, but if exaggeration or flattening occurs, it can put under strain on the surrounding supporting tissues which in turn can cause the pain and stiffness that we know as chronic low back pain.

Lateral plane curves

Ideally, when viewed from behind, the spine should be straight, the hips and shoulders level and the head should face the front without any undue twisting. Once again, unfortunately, this is the exception rather than the rule and all too often lateral plane (side to side) curves develop.

The following list gives the most common causes of this development:

- One leg that is shorter than the other. The difference need only be very slight, at least when you are young and active.
- A broken leg that healed leaving the limb slightly shorter; or a limb that fractured during a growth spurt and was in plaster, so enabling the unaffected leg to grow a little longer.
- One foot that is flat.
- Damage to or the removal of the cartilage of one knee.

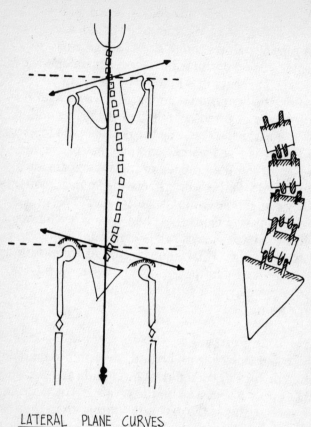

LATERAL PLANE CURVES

- A congenitally shallow or dislocated hip joint.
- A smaller pelvic bone on one side of the hip than the other.
- A large post-operative scar in the abdominal muscles on one side of the body can pull the body over a little to that side.
- An unusual development of one or more vertebrae may give a twist, or scoliosis, to the spine.
- Old broken ribs on one side.
- Long periods of work in which the body is held in one position. Copy typists are a typical example as they may keep their work to one side of their machines all

day long. Over a number of years, the muscles on one side of the spine will build up, so causing a lateral plane curve. This is not so common now with computer typing and the use of word processors and VDUs, but it is likely that these machines too will cause their own problems in the not too distant future.

- People who are blind in one eye or deaf in one ear hold themselves with their good eye or ear forward, so eventually developing a rotation twisting in their spines. Because of the way the spine is built, rotation twisting will always be accompanied by a degree of side bending. The curves will also be carried down the spine so that the body's weight is always brought back into line — this is compensation.

COMPENSATION

As the list above indicates and any osteopath will tell you, 'normal' (or in other words ideal) posture is very rare indeed. But the fact that this does not cause the majority of us any inconvenience is due to the phenomenon known as compensation.

In terms of posture, the body does its utmost to make good any defects by adjusting in other areas, so that if the head is twisted to the left to present a good eye or ear forward, the shoulders are very often twisted to the right to compensate. If the lumbar curve is very pronounced in the final stages of pregnancy, the dorsal spine curve above will probably deepen to compensate (see diagram on page 20). Pregnancy, however, is a relatively short-lived state; the problems really occur when the spine has had a curve for over 20 years.

Given good compensation the body can cope for many years with discs wearing thin. Osteopaths cannot give their patients new backs, but they can find out how best to help the body's own compensation mechanisms. This might involve slightly straightening a curve in one place or

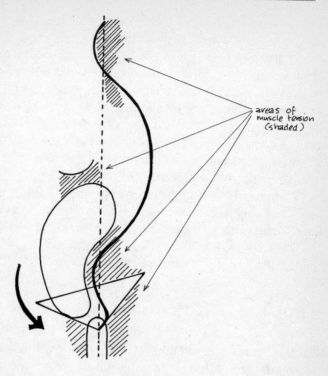

areas of
muscle tension
(shaded)

LUMBAR CURVES IN A HEAVILY PREGNANT WOMAN

even accentuating a curve in another place if that is what
the body demands. It might mean a specific set of
exercises tailor-made for each patient or suggesting ways
of working or playing sport a little differently so that the
spine works to its best mechanical advantage. Very
occasionally a problem will recur no matter what anyone
does for the patient. In such cases the osteopath relieves
the pain as rapidly as possible each time it occurs.

ACUTE SPINAL TRAUMA

To help the back to carry the body's weight, there are
supporting muscles and ligaments. These particular
tissues are among the strongest in the body, but if we

abuse them or treat them badly they will fail and tear or become overstrained.

Back strains usually result from normal activities that are performed incorrectly. In other words we take our backs by surprise. It is not unknown for strong men, who are used to lifting heavy weights, to strain their backs bending to pick up something ridiculously light. This is almost invariably because they took their backs by surprise and made the classic mistake of bending from the waist instead of from the knees.

Injuries also occur in car or sports accidents where forces are applied from outside the body and the shock is taken through the spine before the protecting muscles can contract.

Back strains will heal if properly treated, but if not they can become the focus of trouble for years to come. The scar tissue that forms is rigid and inelastic, unlike the original tissue. Careful osteopathic treatment at the time will allow the body to heal with minimal scar tissue and with all parts of the spine in their correct alignment.

SLIPPED DISC

The discs are pads of fatty tissue that separate the vertebrae in our backs. They receive more blame for acute back pain than any other tissue in the body. This is frequently unfair as they are often the most abused tissues in the body. In fact the slipped or ruptured disc per se is not the main reason for back pain at all.

A typical lumbar disc looks a bit like an onion with a soft jelly-like centre. The layers on the outside of the disc are called the annulus, and the soft centre is called the nucleus.

Each disc is a self-contained fluid system that absorbs shocks. It will only allow a small amount of compression, and owing to fluid displacement within the nucleus some movement can take place. A disc separates the two adjacent vertebrae and prevents them from rubbing on each other. It also prevents pinching or compression of the spinal nerves as they pass out from the spine between the two vertebrae.

ANNULUS FIBROSUS

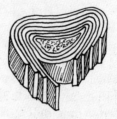

Layer concept
of
annulus fibrosus

Circumferential annular
fibres about the centrally
located pulpy nucleus
(nucleus pulposus)

(vertebra
seen from
below)

The individual discs are firmly bound to the bones above and below and to two thick gristly ligaments in front and behind. These ligaments are known as the anterior and posterior longitudinal ligaments. They run the entire length of the spine, from the top of the neck to the base, and bind the bones and discs together in one long flexible chain. They have many pain-sensitive nerve endings attached to them, especially in the region of each disc. This is why you can tell very quickly if these ligaments have been overstretched or pulled sharply.

The posterior longitudinal ligament gets narrower as it nears the base of the spine, so it cannot protect the discs at the bottom of the spine in the same way that it can higher up. This is why most slipped discs occur near the base of the spine.

Why does a disc slip or rupture?

If too much pressure is put upon a disc, it will fail and tear or break just like any other system in the body. The layers of the annulus, the containing outer case of the disc, will bulge or rupture, allowing the semi-fluid nucleus to leak into the crack created by the bulge. If the outermost layer is still intact it will bulge just like the bulge on the wall of a car tyre. This is known as a disc herniation. It can cause low back ache with pain and stiffness first thing in the morning as the spine takes the body's weight again after being horizontal all night. In fact if you measured yourself first thing in the morning and last thing at night there would be about one centimetre difference. This is because the discs absorb water during the night when the body is not squeezing down on them, and so when you get up the discs are thicker.

If a disc's outer case is damaged the back muscles tighten up to protect the weak disc as it is compressed and so we feel stiff. People with disc problems complain that they cannot bend to put their socks or tights on first thing in the morning, but can bend easily enough to take them off again at night.

Sometimes the trauma is very great and the annulus actually ruptures or splits completely. Then a piece of the

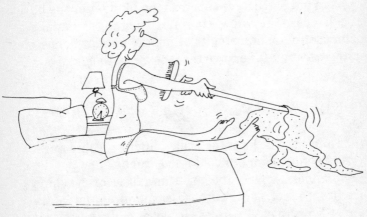

People with disc problems complain they cannot put their socks or tights on first thing in the morning....

soft nucleus is squeezed out of the disc in the way that toothpaste is squeezed out of a tube. If the nucleus comes into contact with one of the nerves that leave the spinal cord between the vertebrae, it can trap or pinch it causing severe pain, numbness or pins and needles down the buttock, leg or even in the foot. The reason why you feel the symptoms so far away from the cause of the pain is because these nerves supply sensation to the areas where it hurts. If the sciatic nerve (the one that runs from the pelvis to the thigh) is the one that is trapped, the condition is known as sciatica.

Most herniated or even ruptured discs do very well without surgical treatment. Osteopaths can help relieve the pressure and muscle spasm of the area, so allowing the disc to heal and become strong again. At first, they will probably prescribe bed rest and treat these patients at home, using gentle stretch techniques so as to allow the bulge to be gradually reabsorbed in its own time. Osteopaths cannot, however, put the disc back. Nobody can. The patient who comes in and is miraculously put right in one treatment as the osteopath cracks his back (see page 63) is not suffering from this type of back problem.

Occasionally, however, the pressure on the nerve root is too strong, or the patient is in danger of losing control of nerves to vital structures such as the bladder or the bowel. In such a case the osteopath refers back to the patient's doctor for an opinion about getting the patient to hospital for an operation to remove the disc altogether.

SPONDYLOSIS (WEAR AND TEAR ARTHRITIS)

Wear and tear of the spine is like paying income tax — most of us just cannot avoid it eventually.

Spondylosis affects the bones and discs of the spine together. In fact, some authorities maintain that a disc cannot rupture or slip unless it has already started to degenerate and wear thin. The bones produce irritating lips or spurs that show up on X-rays as rough edges. Muscles lose their elasticity and become inflexible and therefore are not as efficient at protecting the back against the daily strains of bending and lifting.

However, wear and tear arthritis is not necessarily painful. Most osteopaths agree that if every person over the age of 30 was X-rayed, more than 90 per cent would show some degree of degenerative change in their spine, although the number suffering from backache would be really quite small. The reason for this is because the body compensates for the wear and tear (see page 19).

TENSION AND EMOTIONAL PROBLEMS

Each of us needs a safety valve, a weak link built into our system that acts as an early warning sign of stress and tension. Some people suffer from chronic indigestion and some get alternate diarrhoea or constipation. Some recognise back and neck muscle tension as early warning signs telling them to slow down, in the same way that others get migraine headaches. But what is the link between back pain and stress?

Deep inside our bodies are glands that secrete powerful hormones such as adrenalin which exists, as it does in all primates, to provide a fight or flight response to stress. Unfortunately, unlike animals we cannot always snarl or growl in times of adversity or even run away. Instead we have to bottle up our emotions and hide them for the sake of social convention and in this way the stress is directed inwards. Family problems, financial pressures, sexual fears and self doubts all cause repressed emotions that take their toll on our bodies. If it were possible to accept or display some of these emotional responses, the majority of us would be much happier and a great deal more relaxed. But what generally happens is that our necks and backs get stiff and ache as the pressures mount and once again they either hurt for their own sakes or else a compensation mechanism is disturbed and other muscles and ligaments

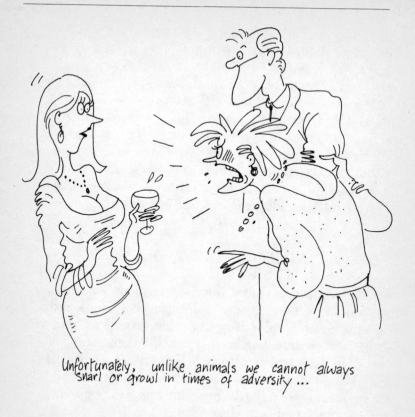

Unfortunately, unlike animals we cannot always snarl or growl in times of adversity ...

have to take the strain.

The osteopath can help relax tired muscles without the need for tranquillisers or pain-killing drugs, but sometimes the patient may need counselling from other agencies to get to the root of a problem outside the scope of osteopathy. The trained osteopath will recognize the symptoms of serious depressive illness or psychological conditions, and will suggest to the patient a source of help for these problems.

OTHER CAUSES OF BACK PAIN

Back pain caused by postural faults, trauma, disc injuries, spondylosis and stress are the commonest back conditions that an osteopath treats. There are many other causes of back pain, however, some of which are outside the scope of osteopathic treatment

- Narrowing of the canal that runs down the spine and carries the spinal cord is called spinal stenosis and can cause severe cramping pain in both legs.
- Ankylosing spondylitis or rheumatoid arthritis are inflammatory conditions of the spine that require hospital treatment to control the disease process. Later, an osteopath might help the body's compensation for the damage that the disease has done, but osteopaths do not treat the inflammation as such, and in fact no properly trained osteopath would treat the acute phase of any inflammatory disease.
- Cancer of the spine (either arising in the spine itself as a primary site or as a secondary site from other places such as the breast or the prostate) is obviously outside an osteopath's care, although it is quite possible for osteopaths to treat the terminally ill (see page 34).
- Sometimes bones become weak and brittle as calcium is lost in conditions such as osteoporosis. In extreme cases the bones fracture. This calcium loss can affect women after their menopause and GPs generally prescribe hormone replacements — oestrogens — together with dietary supplements of calcium to help the bones to become strong and hard again.
- Low back pain can be caused by problems in the pelvic organs or the kidneys. Women who complain of back pain with sexual intercourse may be diagnosed by a gynaecologist as having a tilted womb. But a different bed or lovemaking technique (see pages 76 and 80) may be the only treatment needed.
- Period pain often occurs as low back pain and in such cases osteopathic treatment to improve the drainage of blood from the pelvis can be very helpful.
- People who suffer from chronic constipation often get deep low backache that spreads to the abdominal

muscles or the sides. Here the osteopath might suggest increasing the fibre content of the diet as well as ensuring that the spine is not suffering undue stress, so that the bowel works better and more efficiently.

So you see that what you might think is simple lumbago can have a variety of causes. It might indeed be a simple strain, but it can just as easily be a problem with a much longer history.

3.
THINKING ABOUT OSTEOPATHY

You will probably have many questions to ask before deciding whether to consult an osteopath or not. This chapter will attempt to answer some of them.

Do I really need osteopathy?

No-one needs osteopathy in the way that they need an operation to set a broken leg. No-one actually needs to take an aspirin to relieve a simple headache, but why suffer the pain when there is a reliable alternative?

What is osteopathy?

Briefly, osteopathy is a method of diagnosis and treatment that lays especial emphasis on the body's structural and mechanical problems, but you'll find a fuller discussion of what osteopathy is on pages 9 to 12.

Is it safe?

Osteopathic diagnosis and treatment is almost entirely manual. No drugs are used so there are no problems of harmful side effects. Occasionally an osteopath will prescribe a drug to reduce pain or the inflammation of a joint, but this is always a short-term measure to give the patient relief from acute pain. Although a few osteopaths use electric treatment (page 60), no harsh instruments are used during treatment, because in most cases treatment is with the osteopath's hands. During their thorough and rigorous training all qualified osteopaths are taught never to use force to manipulate or move a patient's joint. If the joint will not move they just use another method — there are hundreds to choose from.

Will it work?

Few forms of treatment have a 100 per cent success rate, and osteopathy certainly doesn't. However, for problems that may be caused by a malfunction of the musculoskeletal system the success rate is very high. Osteopathy cannot cure mumps or measles, but could relieve your nagging back pain. Be guided by the osteopath; you will be told, generally at the end of your first visit (see Chapter 4), whether or not osteopathy is the answer to your problem.

Will the cure be permanent?

This will entirely depend on what took you to the osteopath in the first place. If you have injured a muscle during some sporting activity, the osteopath cannot restore your muscle to its previous healthy condition — no-one can. The body will eventually heal itself, but the osteopath can ensure that it heals in such a way that the damage is minimized (see pages 11 to 12), so that if you continue with the sport the muscle is less likely to break down again.

Is osteopathy preventive? Can it stop me having problems?

No, osteopathy is not preventive. If your body is functioning correctly you do not need osteopathy. However, a large part of an osteopath's work is 'maintenance osteopathy'. Osteopaths cannot turn back the clock and restore their patients to their previous condition, but they can ensure that a problem is contained. This is particularly so with elderly people who find that, say, a regular quarterly visit to the osteopath for treatment to an arthritic joint helps them remain active and independent.

Do I need a letter from my doctor?

No. Osteopaths work as independent practitioners in private practice and do not need a letter of referral from a patient's doctor. In fact many of their patients self-refer, that is they consult the osteopath directly and not via a doctor. If you want your doctor to give you a letter that's fine, but as doctors and osteopaths approach their patients' problems from two quite different viewpoints (see page 47), it is not necessary.

Should I tell my doctor?

That's up to you and will probably depend on your relationship with your doctor. If you only go to the surgery very occasionally it is probably unnecessary. However, if you are a regular patient, and particularly if you've already had treatment for the condition that's taking you to the osteopath, it is certainly courteous to do so.

What if my doctor doesn't think it's a good idea?

Again, it will depend on your opinion of your doctor whether or not you take that advice. But first try to find the reason for the doctor's view, because there are still many GPs who reject any form of treatment that doesn't conform to the medical world in which they were trained.

What if I am on a course of drugs?

The osteopath will ask you this during your first consultation. You won't be expected to stop them, but you may find, particularly if the drugs were used to mask pain, that after a few treatments you may not need them anyway.

What will the osteopath want to know?

On your first visit the osteopath will ask you many questions to build up a picture of your medical history and your way of life (see Chapter 4).

Is there anything I should do before going to the osteopath?

Not really, though it would be helpful to make a note of the precise name and dosage of any drugs you take. It is also sometimes helpful to think about how you will describe your problem and when and how it started. Your appointment with the osteopath will be relaxed and unhurried, but there is no point in wasting time.

Are there any times when I shouldn't go to the osteopath?

The only time an osteopath will advise against treatment is between the 12th and 16th weeks of pregnancy. Spontaneous abortions (miscarriages) are most likely to occur at these times, and while there is absolutely nothing to link osteopathic treatment with having a miscarriage, osteopaths prefer to avoid these times so that if the mother does miscarry she will not feel guilty and have the nagging regret 'If only I hadn't ...'. Osteopathy can be extremely beneficial at other times during pregnancy (see page 91).

How long will the appointments last?

First appointments are usually for an hour, and subsequent ones for 20 to 30 minutes.

How long will the treatment take?

This will depend on your problem. But the osteopath will tell you at the end of the first visit how long the treatment is likely to take.

How much will it cost?

Fees vary, but generally they are in the region of £15 for the first visit and £10 for each subsequent visit. Do not hesitate to ask when making your first appointment as osteopaths expect to be asked that question. And most osteopaths will reduce their fees in cases of genuine need.

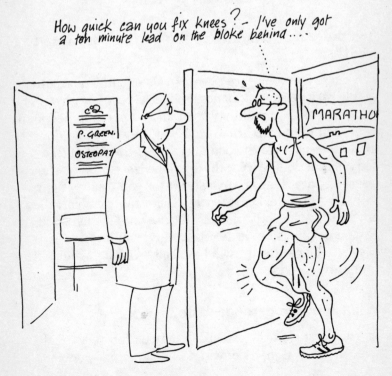

Can I get the fees from medical insurance?

Yes. Some of the bigger medical insurance groups will pay the fees of recognized osteopaths, and the number of osteopaths they recognize is increasing all the time.

Can the osteopath give me a sickness certificate?

Yes. Certificates from qualified osteopaths are accepted by the DHSS and most employers. However, sickness certificates can now be written by the patient.

Does the osteopath just do backs?

No. From the description of osteopathy on page 9 you will realize that osteopaths are concerned with any problem related to the mechanical and structural functioning of the musculoskeletal system of the body.

Are there any conditions the osteopath cannot treat?

Yes, there are a few (see page 27). Osteopaths do not treat people with very weak bones or elderly people with very brittle bones. Nor will they treat an acutely inflamed joint, as in rheumatoid arthritis. However they can, and do, treat other parts of the body because if the rest of the body is functioning well, there will be less strain on the diseased part. This is why osteopaths will treat patients with, for example, heart disease or terminal cancer: they are treating the body, not the disease, and if the rest of the patient's body is made as relaxed and comfortable as possible their suffering will be eased, even though it cannot be cured.

What will the osteopath do?

At your first visit the osteopath may not do very much beyond ask you many questions and examine you very thoroughly. After that you will probably be treated with gentle manipulation and soft tissue massage (see page 61).

Will it hurt?

It might, although this doesn't happen often because osteopathy is a very gentle manipulative treatment and osteopaths are trained never to use force. If the technique they are using is not having the desired effect they change the technique, not apply more force. Occasionally in HVT (see page 63) a patient may experience a brief stab of pain, but it is very brief.

Will I have to undress?

You will be asked to undress to your underclothes — pants for men, bra and pants for women, although swimming trunks or a bikini if you would feel more comfortable in these. The osteopath needs to see as much of you as is decently possible to help in the assessment of your problem (see page 52). If you have a neck or shoulder problem you may only need to undress to the waist.

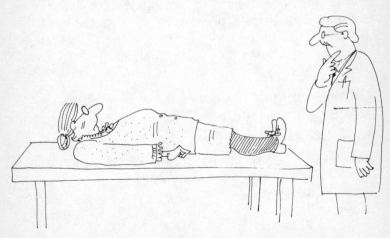

The osteopath has to see as much of you as is decently possible to help in the assessment of your problem...

Will the osteopath come to me?

Yes if you are immobile or in severe pain. A large part of an osteopath's work is in the form of home visits to patients. This, of course, is another advantage of the manual method of treatment — the equipment for the treatment inevitably comes with the osteopath!

How do I find an osteopath?

You can look in the yellow pages telephone directory. But the best way is to write to the General Council and Register of Osteopaths at the address given on page 99, asking for the names and addresses of registered osteopaths in your area. You will then be sure that the osteopaths whose names you receive are properly qualified.

Will the osteopath tell me what my problem is?

At the end of your first visit the osteopath will give you a diagnosis of your problem, in clear simple language. If some words of jargon creep in, ask what they mean — after all it's only fair that you should understand your problem. Very occasionally the osteopath may want you to have some further tests, perhaps an X-ray at the local hospital. But you will be told the reasons for the tests and given the results when they come through.

Will the osteopath know if there is something seriously wrong with me?

Osteopaths receive a thorough training in differential diagnosis (see page 49), precisely so that they can tell if a patient has a problem that cannot be treated osteopathically.

What if the osteopath cannot treat my problem?

If this is the case, the osteopath will immediately refer you back to your GP, or to another appropriate source of help.

What if I don't like the osteopath?

Stop making appointments for treatment; you're under no obligation to continue.

What if I don't think the osteopath is treating me correctly?

Go to another osteopath for a second opinion. If, however, you have any complaint about the professional behaviour of the osteopath, write to the GCRO (address on page 99). Qualified osteopaths are governed by a very strict code of professional ethics and all but the most frivolous complaints are treated very seriously.

What do the initials after an osteopath's name mean?

They indicate where the osteopath trained and his or her professional standing — the full list of initials is on pages 98 to 99.

What is a properly qualified osteopath?

An osteopath who has successfully completed a recognized course of training and so is entitled to use certain of the initials listed on pages 98 to 99 after his or her name.

How do I know if an osteopath is properly qualified?

Look for initials after the name and check what they stand for (pages 98 to 99). If there are no initials stay well clear.

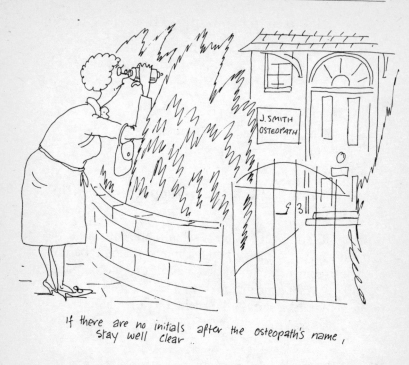

If there are no initials after the osteopath's name, stay well clear..

What is the difference between an osteopath and a physiotherapist?

Briefly, osteopaths are trained to make their own diagnosis of a patient's condition and prescribe and carry out treatment accordingly. Physiotherapists are not trained to do this; instead they must carry out the instructions of the patient's doctor. Unlike osteopaths, physiotherapists use a whole range of mechanical equipment in their treatment of patients. A fuller discussion of the differences is given on pages 92 to 93.

What is the difference between osteopaths and chiropractors?

Chiropractors concentrate on the spine. They use X-rays a great deal to diagnose malfunction and malposition of joints, and their treatment is based on the restoration of function by the repositioning of bones. Osteopaths, on the other hand, use X-rays less frequently, preferring to make their diagnoses by observation and palpation and restore function, i.e. movement, to a joint, by gradually extending the range of movement that joint can make.

What is palpation?

Palpation is feeling with your fingers. It plays a vitally important role in osteopathy as it enables the osteopath to gain an impression of the tissues of the patient's body (see page 53).

What is motion testing?

Exactly what the name says. The osteopath tests the ability of a joint to move by moving it (see page 54).

What is HVT?

HVT stands for High Velocity Thrust, sometimes called 'bone cracking' — though rarely by osteopaths! You'll find a fuller description of this form of osteopathic treatment on page 63.

What is cranial osteopathy

Cranial osteopathy is a specialised form of osteopathy. It follows the teachings of William Garner Sutherland, a student of Dr Still the founder of osteopathy. Dr Sutherland discovered that the bones of the skull move and are not fixed as they appear to be when you see an ancient skull. They move with the help of an extremely complicated system of flanges and bevelled joints. The degree of movement is very small, but the bones can be palpated by highly trained osteopaths.

The brain is contained inside the skull and is bathed with cerebrospinal fluid. This fluid is secreted in the brain and flows down and out of the skull to bathe the complete spinal cord and the roots of the spinal nerves. The brain is suspended within the skull by sheets of tissue known as meninges and fascia held under tension. Long sheets of the fascia pass down through the large hole at the base of the skull (the foramen magnum), form the lining of the spinal canal and are finally attached to the sacrum at the base of the vertebral column. (The sacrum is the large flat bone situated between the large pelvic bones on either side of the body.)

Practitioners of cranial osteopathy maintain that there is a rhythmical pulsation, distinct from the respiratory rhythm or the pulse of the cardiovascular system, which pumps the cerebrospinal fluid and which can be felt by minute pressure on the skull bones or at the sacrum as well as elsewhere in the body. This is the so-called cranial rhythm. Each cranial bone moves along a set axis guided by its articulation with its neighbours and any disturbance of normal cranial bone motion will lead to disturbances of normal cranial rhythm and thus disturbance of normal tissue fluid flow.

Cranial treatment, which is an extremely gentle technique, tries to balance the rhythmical forces at work in the body by gently guiding and releasing the tensions within the tissues. It is good for problems that relate directly to the head, such as migraine, sinusitis and trauma.

This technique is particularly suitable for children, or nervous or tense adults who may respond better to this passive involuntary approach rather than to direct or thrust treatment. But not all osteopaths give this treatment as it is not included in the curriculum of all the training schools. It is therefore very important, if this is the type of treatment you think you need, to make sure that the practitioner you wish to consult practises it.

What is visceral osteopathy?

One of the basic tenets of osteopathic philosophy is that movement is essential to the body's normal growth and repair. If a state exists where this normal movement is inhibited, it follows that normal organ function cannot take place. This has been the basis of osteopathic treatment of visceral (organ) disease for many years. Orthodox medicine has long held these views in scant regard, because orthodox medicine has been based in modern times on the germ theory of disease.

Now, however, research programmes in the USA are validating the osteopathic view. Professor Irwin Korr of the Texas College of Osteopathic Medicine is one of a number of prominent workers in this field. He has written extensively on the reflex (automatic) pathways that exist between the nervous system and the organs and maintains that the reflexes can exist in both directions — from organ to muscle and from muscle to organ. He has also shown that proteins can pass down the nerves from the spinal cord to the organs via these reflex pathways, and if there is a block in normal reflex pathways, the organ can suffer and eventually dysfunction.

Osteopaths treat patients with problems in the cardiovascular system, the gastric system, the respiratory system, and the reproductive system to name a few. But remember that it is not the disease that is being treated, but the body that houses the disease. Osteopaths seek to

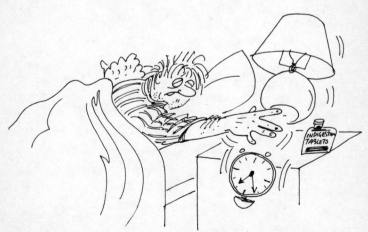

The next time you reach for an indigestion tablet remember that there could be another way of treating this problem.

create a better environment so the body can adapt to change and return to normal functioning.

This is not to say that all disease states are amenable to osteopathic treatment — they are not and it would be foolish to pretend otherwise. However, the next time you reach for an indigestion tablet or a painkiller for your period pain, remember that there could be another way of treating the problem.

4.
YOUR FIRST VISIT TO THE OSTEOPATH

Most people's first visit to the osteopath is prompted by
back pain. And we have all heard of someone who had
their 'disc put back' after only one visit and so had been
miraculously cured after years of pain. How nice if such
stories were really true! What may seem a miracle to the
patient is, in fact, the result of the osteopath's careful
observation, examination and questioning of the patient.
This enables the osteopath to build up a picture of the
patient and his or her way of life, which is extremely
important in making a correct diagnosis and prescribing
the right treatment. That is why your first visit may seem
little more than a question and answer session.

This chapter gives a general picture of what to expect
the first time you visit the osteopath, although there may
be slight variations and differences from one osteopath
to another.

BEFORE THE VISIT

When you've made an appointment to see an osteopath (see page 35 for details of how to find qualified osteopaths in your area), make a note of any drug or other form of treatment that you are having. The osteopath will find it helpful to know the name of the drug, the dosage and how long you have been taking it. Make a note, too, of any herbal or homeopathic remedies you take regularly. All this will help the osteopath and ensure that none of the appointment is wasted while you try to remember this information.

It is also helpful to jot down points about the problem which is forcing you to seek an osteopath's help. For example, when did it start, is the pain constant, or does it get worse after exertion or when you are tired.

THE PRELIMINARY QUESTIONS

The osteopath will start the diagnostic procedure the moment you walk into the consulting room — age, sex, physical build, the way you move and so on. These observations give the osteopath a basic idea of anything that can safely and automatically be ruled out — a man is not going to be suffering from a gynaecological problem and a child of four or five is unlikely to be suffering from osteoarthritis.

Some osteopaths have their receptionists take down information such as the patient's name, address, age and so on, others prefer to do this themselves. It is entirely a matter of the individual osteopath's preference.

Once these details are dealt with, the osteopath will need to have some background information about you. The questions will cover such topics as age, career, marital status, number of children, leisure activities, are you fit for your age and so on. If you look older than your years, this could be a clue to general unhealthiness or a sign of considerable stress in your life.

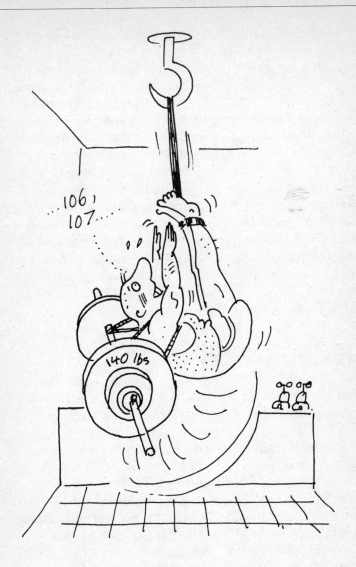

...people do amazing things to their bodies to keep fit...

Your weight and height will be recorded and the osteopath will ask if the former has changed much recently. Your job will provide clues here. For example a change from an active to a sedentary office job could well cause changes in weight. The change might even be the reason why you are consulting the osteopath.

The osteopath needs to know about your leisure activities because people do amazing things to their bodies to keep fit and for the sake of sport. The behaviour of many sportsmen and women borders on the obsessional, which makes treating the almost inevitable injuries difficult. So the osteopath is not being nosey when asking about how you spend your leisure, but is seeking clues to causes. After all, if you spend your weekends hunched over a chessboard, your problems are unlikely to be the same as if you had sprinted around an athletics track or played a hard game of tennis.

THE PATIENT'S STORY

After the preliminary questions are over the osteopath will turn to your specific problem — the reason why you are there.

You will usually be asked a very general, leading question, such as 'How can I help you?' or 'What brings you here today?'. Such a question is the cue for you to describe, in your own words, the problem that has caused you to seek the osteopath's help. Do not worry if you feel your description is long-winded or that you are not expressing yourself very clearly. Relax, take your time. Osteopaths work in private practice. They see their patients on an appointment basis, usually allowing 20 to 30 minutes for each treatment and up to an hour for a first visit. Therefore the waiting-room outside is not full of other anxious people.

You will be asked to point out where the pain is, and this in itself can be quite revealing to the osteopath. A line of pain might indicate a nerve root, a whole area of pain might stem from a structure deep within the body. The adjectives used to describe your symptoms are also useful clues — constricting or burning pain is different from throbbing or toothache-type pain.

The nature and timing of pain is very important to the osteopath in building up a picture of your problems. Cardiac pain is often a constricting or crushing pain in the chest that radiates up into the left side of the neck or down into the left arm and is immediately made worse with exertion. On the other hand disc problems often produce low back ache and stiffness that seems worst first thing in the morning, to such an extent that putting on socks or tights is extremely difficult. If you had mild sciatica you could probably walk for about 20 minutes without too much discomfort in the leg, but if you were suffering from hardening of the arteries you might get severe calf pain after only half a mile.

If you think that these questions are very similar to those your doctor would ask, this is not really the case. All the time the osteopath is looking at the function of your whole body and how your life with the pain has changed. The osteopath wants to find out about the patient before the onset of the pain in order to assess why the pain came on. Your doctor, on the other hand, has been trained from a very different viewpoint. Instead of looking at the whole structure, as an osteopath does, a doctor looks for symptoms and tries to fit them into patterns or syndromes. The physical tests made by a doctor during the examination of a patient are designed to confirm these views.

THE DETAILED QUESTIONS

Once you have described your problem and its symptoms in as much detail as you can, the osteopath will go through a series of detailed questions to find out which tissue is at fault and what that fault might be. That key phrase in osteopathy — structure governs function — lies behind the osteopath's questions as the means of obtaining the necessary clues to the cause of your problem.

Each tissue in the body will behave in a certain way under certain conditions. Using this knowledge the osteopath asks questions that implicate one tissue or another, because each tissue can be in pain for a different reason. For example a joint can be affected by trauma, an infection, a tumour, inflammation or simply by changes due to the body's natural ageing process.

Though the osteopath may ask the same question, your answers will vary according to the cause of the problem. If you have pain on movement this might implicate a muscle guarding a painful joint rather than a nerve, yet heat will make a tense muscle relax while the same heat will make an infected joint worse. If you have pain in the ribs, this might be caused by a muscular problem or by pleurisy involving the lining of the lung. If you have pleurisy you will not have a history of trauma to the rib area, whereas if your problem is muscular you will not have the signs and symptoms of a lung infection. The two conditions are quite different and so your answers to the same questions will be different.

These are just a few examples of the sort of questions that you may be asked and are used to illustrate how the osteopath thinks and the reasons for all the questions — some of which might otherwise seem rather irrelevant.

Having dealt with the matter of individual tissues, the osteopath will want to know the history of your problem and what, if any, treatment you have had. Have you seen the doctor and was any medication prescribed? A very common question is whether your doctor knows you are going to see an osteopath. GPs, on the whole, are now quite well disposed to osteopaths and very often refer the patient with a covering letter. Have you had any blood tests or X-rays and if so does your GP have the results? Most doctors are quite cooperative about releasing this sort of information to the osteopath with your permission.

At the first visit, the osteopath will take a detailed medical case history just like your doctor. This is necessary because osteopaths work independently of doctors or hospitals and see patients who refer themselves.

Mechanical pain can mimic serious problems and if the osteopath were not thoroughly trained in diagnosing the difference between one sort of pain and another — what is known as a differential diagnosis — then serious mistakes could occur. However a fully trained osteopath spends four years training to differentially diagnose problems, so you can be confident that mistakes very rarely occur. But it is for this reason that a full and frank account of your past and present medical history forms an essential part of your first visit to the osteopath. Some patients are simply not suitable for treatment for one reason or another (page 27) and these questions about past health are essential if such patients are to be identified quickly.

Any accidents that you have had in the past can have a bearing on the present problem. Old limb fractures can

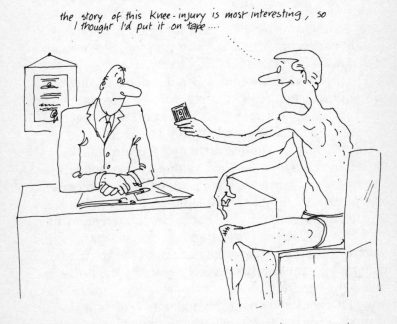

the story of this Knee-injury is most interesting, so I thought I'd put it on tape ....

A full and frank account of your past and present medical history forms an essential part of your first visit to an osteopath ..

cause shortening of the limb or wasting of the muscles involved. Over a long period these can alter someone's posture and eventually lead to the development of a structural fault. The presence of deep scar tissue can mean that the part of the body concerned has lost its elasticity and so cannot readily adapt to change in response to increased mechanical demand. This may be the reason why the body broke down when it did, causing the muscle to go into spasm or the joint to be overstrained. An old football injury to the knee cartilage can mean that in years to come the knee does not work so well and is predisposed to wear and tear and osteoarthritis.

These are all examples to show that we are the product of what has gone before in our lives. It does not mean that every time a child falls over or you are injured on the sports field it is an immediate cause for future concern. But it does mean that if a tissue breaks down today, the forces both within and outside that tissue have had strain patterns built into them depending on what has happened to them in the past. So, just as an osteopath needs to know how you spend your time at work and play, it is also vital to understand the history of your injuries to be able to diagnose and treat them effectively.

You will also be asked detailed questions about your present medical history. During training osteopaths learn all about each of the body's systems and their specific diseases. You will be asked about your respiratory, cardiovascular, gastrointestinal and genito-urinary systems. The reason for this, as already mentioned, is that any system can give what appears to be mechanical aches and pains, and unless the osteopath asks it will be impossible to discover what should be treated and what should be left alone. For example, you might have pain in your side that radiates to the back or to the groin. Such pain may be caused by your kidneys or by the psoas muscle on the front of your spine. However, unless the osteopath asks you about the functioning of your urinary system, including frequency, colour and pain associated with passing water, there is no way that the source of the pain can be identified.

Simple questions about your drinking and smoking habits can be revealing in themselves or act as clues to understanding deeper disease processes, or your overall lifestyle. Questions about recent weight loss or gain, as well as questions about dietary or eating habits will reveal much about your general health.

Finally, the osteopath will want to know about any drugs or medication that you are taking, either prescribed or bought over the counter at the chemist or the health food shop. People think that the words 'drug' and 'medicine' refer only to those their doctor has given them. This is not so. Vitamins or minerals, laxatives or herbal preparations can be just as important as items obtained on prescription.

Osteopaths are not against the use of tablets when the need arises. For example, your osteopath might advise you to take a preparation to reduce inflammation or pain for a short time if the effect will be a beneficial adjunct to your treatment. Osteopaths are trained to look for the more common side effects of common preparations that their patients might be taking. The potential dangers of powerful drugs are very relevant to osteopathy and so most osteopaths have an up-to-date text book on drugs or will telephone the local chemist if in doubt about a particular preparation.

By now the osteopath will have built up a detailed picture about you, the tissue causing your symptoms and the way all this fits into the general pattern of your health, past and present. But without a physical examination, this picture is obviously incomplete.

THE PHYSICAL EXAMINATION

You may not realize it on your first visit, but the physical examination the osteopath will give you follows a series of set procedures. These are observation, palpation and motion testing. Usually you will be examined standing, then sitting and finally lying down, although there may well be some variations to this overall pattern.

THE STANDING EXAMINATION

Observation

This quite simply involves the osteopath looking at you, first as a whole and then at the specific part that is in trouble. This enables the osteopath to see the connection between the two.

You will usually be asked to undress to your underclothes, bra and pants for women and pants for men, though you could wear a swimsuit or a bikini if you felt more comfortable in that. The reason for undressing is that the osteopath needs to see as much of you as is practical and decent to be able to evaluate your local problem within the context of your whole body function. To understand how the lumbar spine performs and therefore got into trouble, the osteopath needs to see the hips and the legs as well as the rest of the spine. However, if you just have a neck or a shoulder problem, it may only be necessary to strip to the waist (leaving the bra on if you are a woman). Some osteopaths have a special back fastening gown for their patients to wear, but this is the exception rather than the rule.

The osteopath will examine you first from behind. You will be assessed for the effect of gravity on your frame as you stand upright. If you are in so much pain that the very act of standing is impossible, the osteopath will proceed directly to the sitting or lying down examinations. Assuming, though, that you can stand comfortably for even a few minutes, the osteopath starts by looking for your 'normal' postural curves, and the presence or absence of the side to side curves (see pages 17 to 19). Using various anatomical landmarks, such as the level of your head and shoulders, the position of your shoulder blades, waist-folds, cleft of your buttocks, and the apparent length of your legs, the osteopath makes a free-

hand sketch on your record card or chart of exactly how
you are standing without support.

You will be asked to turn to face the side and the
observations will be repeated. From this position the
osteopath notes the carriage of your head, the height of
your chest or bust and the tone of your abdominal
muscles, as well as the front to back curves of your spine.
Again, the osteopath will probably make a free-hand
sketch, as these are very helpful at subsequent visits,
because they will show immediately if your posture has
changed.

Palpation

Next the osteopath will examine you by means of
palpation. To palpate something is to feel it with your
hands. In this context palpation means using the hands to
gain an impression of the tissues, both superficial and
deep, as a part of the diagnostic process. Palpation forms
a major part of the osteopath's examination, because
osteopaths believe that the palpable change in a tissue can
affect the way that tissue functions. They use this fact to
help diagnose the change in the tissue that either caused
the change in its function or, in turn, was itself caused by
the change in function. An osteopath's hands are
diagnostic instruments as well as treatment tools.

The osteopath will palpate your tissues as you are
standing, sitting and lying down. Again, the first part of
the examination is global — you will feel the osteopath's
hands running lightly over your spine and the extremities
of your body to determine the tone and temperature of the
more superficial tissues. Even structures close to the skin
will feel 'ropey' or 'boggy' if there is a local problem.
Sometimes the skin feels warm to the touch or dry like
parchment. Deeper palpation may reveal tissues that are
harder to the touch or tender at specific points. Any pain
or reaction to the pressure may provide a clue as to the
origin of the pain.

Once your whole body has been examined in this way,
the osteopath will palpate the local symptomatic tissues

in a similar manner. After this comes movement testing.

Movement testing

Movement testing is exactly what the phrase suggests — the osteopath will watch and feel you as you move. First the osteopath will ask you to make a particular movement to observe how you do it, then you will be asked to repeat the movement while the osteopath palpates the tissue as it moves. This is active movement testing.

Then, when you stand, sit or lie down, the osteopath will move your body, feeling its response to the movement. This is passive movement testing.

Although other practitioners, such as doctors and physiotherapists, use both active and passive movement testing, it is osteopaths who use it most extensively. They are interested not only in the range or quantity of movement, but also in the quality of that movement. Different structures will inhibit movement in different ways. For example, in the apparently simple movement of bending forward, muscle spasm will inhibit the movement before it gets started if it is protecting a weak disc, while a fibrotic muscle will allow movement but will stop it sooner than expected. By feeling your spine as you bend, first actively and then passively, the osteopath compares the movement obtained with the movement expected and so begins to appreciate more than just the range of movement alone.

While you are standing up, the osteopath will probably ask you to bend forwards, backwards, side to side from left to right, and to rotate your neck or trunk to the left and right. If the osteopath is examining one of your peripheral joints, such as a shoulder or a knee joint, the same tests will be used.

There are many other movements that you may be asked to make. No matter which ones you have to do, the principles are the same. It is movement and the response to that movement by the tissues that is all important to an osteopathic diagnosis.

THE SITTING EXAMINATION

After completing all these tests, the osteopath will ask you to sit down. The same examinations will then be repeated for the osteopath to see how your body responds to them in a seated position. This is particularly important if you have a sedentary occupation.

THE EXAMINATION LYING DOWN

Finally you will be examined lying down — on your stomach, your back and on each side. The tests will be much the same as before, but obviously you cannot bend forward to touch your toes if you are lying on your stomach.

Do not worry if you do not have exactly the same tests as friends who have been to an osteopath. There are no hard and fast rules. Some osteopaths will never examine a shoulder problem with the patient lying down, others always do. It is usually a matter of how the osteopath was trained rather than a reflection on the completeness of the examination or the seriousness of your problem.

OTHER TYPES OF TEST

Orthopaedic testing
Osteopaths are also trained to use standard orthopaedic tests, so your peripheral joints, such as the hips and the knees, will be examined in the same way that your doctor does. Once again, the osteopath will use observation, palpation and active and passive movement testing to help reveal any problems in your peripheral joints that may, or may not, be important to the diagnosis of your problem.

Tests for extra information
Sometimes, after making all these tests, the osteopath

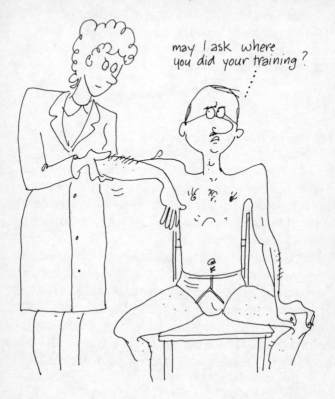

needs more information to complete the diagnosis. All osteopaths are trained to use apparatus to test blood pressure, to use a stethoscope to examine the chest and to use a patella hammer, cotton wool and a pin to examine the nervous system. These tests, as well as others, such as blood tests and urine tests, will help confirm information already obtained. These tests may not form the diagnosis in themselves, but they can provide valuable information that eventually fits into the total diagnostic picture.

If the osteopath needs more information, such as X-rays or blood tests, to rule out disease or its symptoms, this is usually done privately. But you will be given the reasons for the tests, and when the results come through you will either be referred back to your doctor with a covering letter from the osteopath, or your diagnosis will be completed and your osteopathic treatment will begin.

THE DIAGNOSIS

At the end of the examination the osteopath should have some idea of what is wrong with you.

An osteopathic diagnosis is like a story — it has a beginning, a middle and an end. The beginning is the aetiology (why the problem occurred), together with the predisposing factors (why it occurred to you in particular). Next comes the identification of the tissue causing the symptoms and the pathology, in other words what hurts and what has happened to make it hurt. Lastly there is the prognosis or what the osteopath expects to happen as a result of the prescribed treatment.

On your record card the osteopath could well write: 'A short right leg has predisposed the patient to increased wear of the last two lumbar discs on that side. Under normal circumstances she copes well, but as she attempted to lift two particularly heavy shopping bags she overstrained her already overworked muscles and so tore some fibres of the last lumbar disc. She now has acute muscle spasm in the lumbar spine and sciatica due to pressure on the first sacral nerve root as it leaves the spine at the damaged level.'

This is a very typical osteopathic diagnosis for patients of both sexes. In a man the problem is most usually caused by picking up an unusually heavy weight, or something that is quite heavy but in an awkward, difficult to get at place, or over-enthusiastic DIY concrete-laying or similar heavy work. But don't worry, the osteopath will not use this language when explaining your problem to you. Instead you may well be told that your sciatica is due to pressure on the nerve where it leaves the spine because of the recent strain to the back in that area.

The diagnosis is completed by proposing short- and

long-term treatment programmes. At this point in the consultation, you will usually be given an idea of the expected progress of your condition, how many treatments you are likely to need and when to book your next appointment.

YOUR FIRST TREATMENT

The short-term 'first aid' treatment is generally started immediately to help relieve your pain. You could be given some traction and gentle stretching to relieve the nerve root pressure and muscle spasm. In the case outlined in the diagnosis above, bed rest and some tablets to relieve the pain and inflammation would probably also be prescribed.

LONG-TERM TREATMENT

Later, as recovery takes place and you become more mobile as pressure on the nerve root subsides, the osteopath may use some specific manipulation to release the small spinal facet joints that often become locked as a sequel to this problem. Also, to prevent the problem recurring, the osteopath will probably start some work to correct the original postural fault.

5.
THE SECOND VISIT AND OSTEOPATHIC TREATMENTS

Sometimes, one visit to the osteopath is all you will need. An acute strain to the facet joints, those small spinal joints already mentioned, produces a fierce muscle spasm and accompanying pain. If seen quickly enough, work on the affected muscle plus a simple manipulation to break the local locking of the joints means that a 'cure' is effected quite dramatically.

Unfortunately most people do not visit the osteopath soon enough, so that a course of treatment lasting many weeks or even months is needed to ease the painful problem and remedy the underlying cause.

Each time you visit the osteopath the situation is reassessed. You will be carefully questioned about how the tissues are coping with the pain and how you are responding to the previous treatment. It is often quite difficult to judge the amount of treatment that each patient needs at each visit, and you may have an unwanted or painful reaction. These are rare as osteopathic treatment taken as a whole is gentle and relaxing, but that is why careful attention is paid to the effects of the previous treatment. It will also help the osteopath if you keep a note of any reactions, good or bad, to the previous treatment, as this will enable the osteopath to judge how much or how little force you need at each visit to produce the desired effect.

The osteopath will probably explain to you that the progress of your treatment from visit to visit is always judged in the light of the prognosis made at the first visit. At first it may not appear obvious to you that you are getting better, but once you realize that the change in your tissues that led to the problem took many years to become apparent, you will understand that quick change is both unlikely and undesirable. Indeed, particularly in elderly people, there may well be no cure. But, on the other hand, osteopathy can often help contain the problem, so ensuring the patient a healthier and happier old age. And in the same way sports enthusiasts may well be able to keep on with their sport if they have regular maintenance osteopathy to prevent the problem becoming worse.

Every patient an osteopath sees is different, so individual treatment programmes are arranged and prescribed for each patient. At each treatment session various techniques will be used as you lie in different positions on the treatment table. The reason why you are put into the different positions is so that the osteopath can apply the right amount of force or leverage to get the tissue to change under his or her hands. No one technique is applied to any one tissue. Muscle, for example, can be made to relax using rhythmical massage techniques, articulation or stretch techniques, high velocity thrust or 'cracking' techniques. The position you are put in depends on the technique the osteopath is going to use.

Most osteopaths use just their hands for treatment. However, some modern osteopaths recognize that the use of ultrasound machines or electrical apparatus for short-wave diathermy, to relax muscles or reduce inflammation can play a valuable part in osteopathic treatment.

SOFT TISSUE MASSAGE

Soft tissue massage (see diagram on page 62) is exactly what the name implies — massage of the softer tissues of the body. To the untrained eye these techniques look very much like the sort of basic massage that you might receive at a health club or beauty salon. However it is not as simple as that, because the way that the technique is performed can change the effect that the massage has on the tissues concerned.

It is done to skin, fascia (the connective tissue between the skin and underlying muscle) and muscle, depending on the pressure and speed at which it is applied. It can be light or heavy, fast or slow, superficial or deep. It can stimulate tissues, encouraging them to tighten up if they are loose, or it can be soothing to make them relax if they are tight. It can go across a muscle or along its length and is often the starting point in a typical treatment. Above all it is usually pleasant and calming and in fact some patients almost fall asleep during soft tissue massage.

Sometimes an effleurage or draining technique is used if there is excess tissue fluid in a congested area. This technique involves very light stroking movements applied rhythmically to the most superficial structures in that area to drain the lymph channels nearest to the skin. Oil or talc is sometimes used as a lubricant during this procedure to avoid burning or abraiding the skin.

ARTICULATION TECHNIQUES

Articulation techniques are refined passive movement techniques in which the osteopath tries to stretch tissues along their length by gently putting a force along them using either one or a combination of levers. This sounds very complicated, but in practice it just means that the osteopath uses your arm or leg as a lever when applying a gentle force. This use of leverage means that the osteopath has to use less force and therefore less pressure, so making

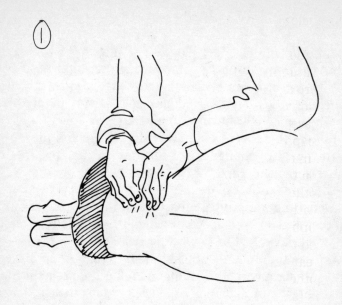

SOFT TISSUE
MASSAGE

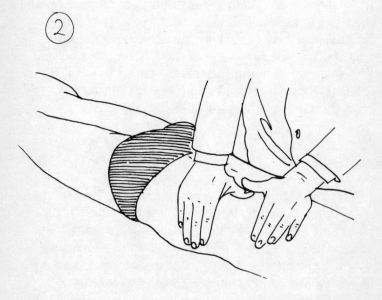

the whole process more controlled and less painful for the patient.

Traction to the shoulder joint is another example of articulation technique. Here the osteopath uses gentle pressure along the arm to encourage separation of the two halves of the shoulder joint. This can be very helpful in such cases as frozen shoulder.

Osteopaths also use manual spinal traction (see diagram on page 64) as opposed to mechanical spinal traction that is commonly found in a hospital's physiotherapy department. In the manual system the osteopath can feel the body's response to the treatment as it is applied and so knows immediately when the body has reached the point of change, thus ensuring it is neither overtreated nor undertreated.

Another form of articulation is called springing the tissues (see diagram on page 65). Here the osteopath literally gently pushes the individual bones with a varying springing pressure so as to stretch the structures between them. Once again, however, it is the feedback obtained through palpation that enables the osteopath to gauge the amount of force required to effect change — neither too much nor too little.

THE HIGH VELOCITY THRUST (HVT)

This technique (see diagrams on pages 66, 67 and 68) is otherwise known as cracking or manipulating the spine, and is probably what most people mistakenly regard as osteopathic treatment. The reasons for the technique's magical reputation is that the results can be dramatic. The patient hears a snap or crack and thinks that the bone or disc has gone back into place. Nothing could be further from the truth. Bones cannot pop out and back in again. If they did they would be dislocating and that would be a case for the orthopaedic surgeon not the osteopath. What actually happens is much more simple.

The boney joints of the body are under a slight vacuum.

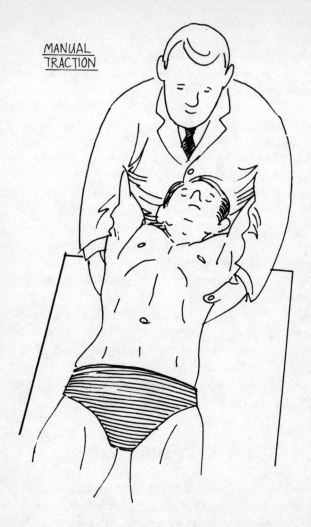

MANUAL TRACTION

When the two surfaces are separated the vacuum is released causing an audible pop — like pulling a rubber sucker away from a wall. However, as the joints separate the nerves of the capsule covering the joint relay information to the spinal cord, registering the fact that the capsule has been slightly stretched. The spinal cord responds by reflexly relaxing the muscles surrounding the joint. It is this that is responsible for the so-called 'miracle cure', because it means that the pain accompanying the

SPRINGING THE TISSUES

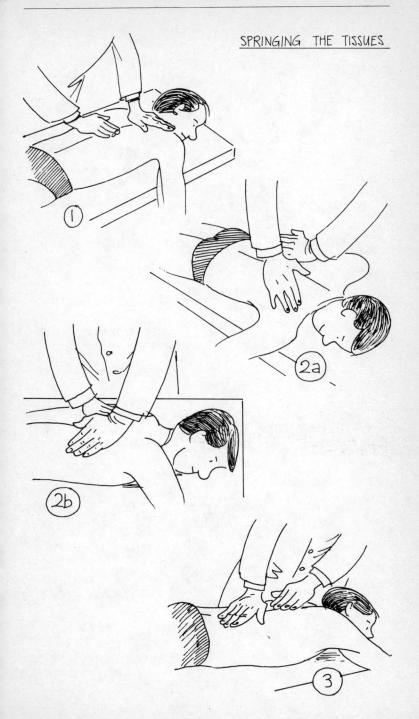

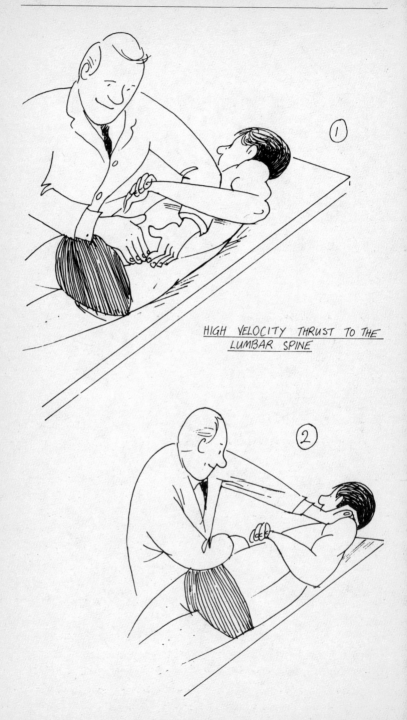

HIGH VELOCITY THRUST TO THE LUMBAR SPINE

muscle spasm goes and there is an appreciable increase in the range of movement now possible. 'One minute I was bent over and the next I was upright and walked out smiling.' In fact, the truth is that the thrust technique is nothing more than a tool that the osteopath uses to effect a change in tight muscles that cannot be relaxed by soft tissue massage techniques because they are too deep. It is a quick and efficient technique, but not applicable in every case.

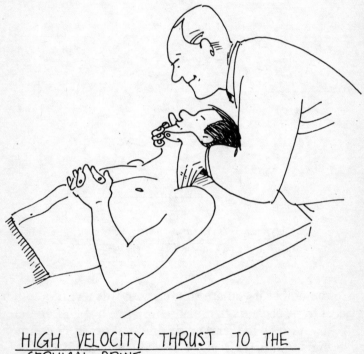

HIGH VELOCITY THRUST TO THE CERVICAL SPINE

It is also a technique that osteopathy students practice on each other long before they are permitted to use it on patients. No properly trained osteopath uses undue force when attempting to manipulate a joint, because force hides ignorance. If a joint will not move with minimum force then another technique is used. The thrust, when it is used, is gentle but firm and usually very fast. It should also be relatively painless although some patients do cry out or grunt, but this is more an involuntary gasp as their chests are momentarily compressed. Any pain or discomfort that does occur lasts for just a split second.

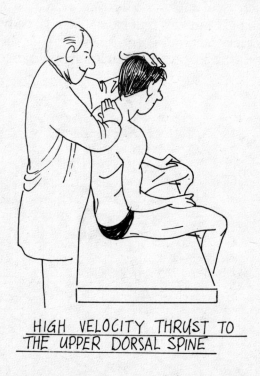

HIGH VELOCITY THRUST TO
THE UPPER DORSAL SPINE

Do remember if you are treated with this technique that it takes three seconds to crack your joint, but half an hour to treat you. Its what goes on during that other 29 minutes 57 seconds that is the real essence of osteopathic treatment.

INVOLUNTARY TECHNIQUES

Osteopaths use involuntary techniques to try to 'destress' tense tissues. Sometimes they are called functional techiques and sometimes they are called cranial techniques (see page 38).

They are extremely gentle passive movement techniques that rely on a very fine sense of palpation. They are usually combined with breathing and so are often used on structures such as the diaphragm, although they can be used all over the body.

The osteopath attempts gently to guide the tissues of the painful or disfunctional part through a series of pathways to reduce the tension. Then, combining a series of these pathways, attempts are made to find a balance point in the tissues where all the stress and force acting on the tissues is minimal. These techniques are so gentle that often the patient drops off to sleep during the treatment and they are especially good with nervous patients or children.

6.
HOW CAN I HELP MYSELF?

Although osteopathy is not intended as a treatment regime solely for sufferers of minor muscular or skeletal problems, it is true that more than 70 per cent of first visits to the osteopath are prompted by low back and neck problems. Many's the patient who has asked 'Could I have done anything to avoid this? Is there anything I can do to stop it happening again?' The answer to the first question is 'Probably not', but to the second it could well be 'Very possibly'. This chapter, therefore, deals with what you can do to help yourself avoid situations which demand too much of your musculoskeletal system, so that acute painful episodes will be less frequent and, when they do occur, short-lived.

COPING WITH THE ACUTE ATTACK

The most important thing to be understood about pain is that it is nature's way of telling you that something is wrong. Acute pain of any sort should never be hidden or ignored. The attitude of 'grin and bear it' is dangerous; if you do not listen to your body when it tells you that you have done wrong, you will repeat the trauma and make any damage that has occurred worse. By listening to your pain, and obeying your body if it indicates you should rest or lie down, your recovery will be quicker and more effective.

Beyond 'Follow the prompting of your body', there are no hard and fast do's and don'ts. Some people with a disc problem feel the need to rest, while others with pain in a similar place cannot stay in one position for too long without fidgeting, because the cause of the pain is different.

Heat or cold
The use of local heat, in the form of hot water bottles or electrical heat pads, is very soothing. Heat lamps, however, are not really suitable as they cannot be used for longer than ten minutes or so without the risk of burning the skin. They are also difficult to position accurately, especially in the neck area.

Some people find cold more effective than heat. In this case use a small packet of frozen peas which is easily moulded to the affected area. It is also less messy than ice cubes wrapped in a towel and is reusable, though don't eat the thawed out peas! Ice is usually best for peripheral injuries to the arms and legs.

Painkillers
Pain-killing drugs or drugs to reduce inflammation can be helpful if they are prescribed and carefully used. The problems occur when patients visit the chemist, dose themselves with powerful painkillers and then return to work, especially if it was the work that caused them to hurt themselves in the first place. Nor should such drugs be taken for too long; analgesics should be a short-term crutch and not a long-term walking stick.

Corsets

During an acute attack of back pain you might find the use of a corset helpful. However, the use of such a support should only be short-term otherwise your muscles can become soft and flabby as they lose tone because their natural supporting role is being taken up by the corset. For a similar reason the lighter weight corsets are better than the very rigid ones. Women sometimes find that an ordinary pantie girdle can be quite helpful.

Collars

Collars, too, are very useful as a short-term aid if you are suffering from acute neck or arm pain. They can be prescribed by your doctor or fitted by the physiotherapy department at your local hospital. It is also both easy and cheap to make your own from tubular bandage and upholstery foam (the diagram on page 73 shows you how to do this).

HOW TO MAKE A SIMPLE COLLAR

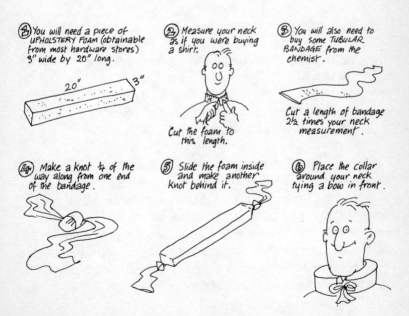

(1) You will need a piece of UPHOLSTERY FOAM (obtainable from most hardware stores) 3" wide by 20" long.

20"   3"

(2) Measure your neck as if you were buying a shirt.

Cut the foam to this length.

(3) You will also need to buy some TUBULAR BANDAGE from the chemist.

Cut a length of bandage 2½ times your neck measurement.

(4) Make a knot ¼ of the way along from one end of the bandage.

(5) Slide the foam inside and make another knot behind it.

(6) Place the collar around your neck tying a bow in front.

Getting out of bed

When you are suffering an acute attack of low back pain, even everyday activities, such as getting in and out of bed or getting up from a chair, can be very painful unless done carefully. The obvious answer is to avoid getting up unless you have to, but if you need to get up, to go to the toilet for example, the following tips might help.

- If you are in bed try and lie on your side; if you have a painful side, it should be uppermost. If this means that you will be facing the wall, move the pillows to the other end of the bed before you lie down.
- Bring your knees up very slowly until the sides of your feet are balanced on the edge of the bed.
- With one hand and one elbow supporting your weight, gently lever yourself up into a sitting position, being very careful not to bend your back at all. If you're not on your own, some help at this stage could be useful. Once in the sitting position, use both arms locked straight at the elbow to support yourself while you move your bottom to the edge of the bed.
- Now put both hands behind you and support your back as you use your legs to stand up. Again try to keep the back straight. You will find that this is much easier with help, and if you keep your feet well apart with one in front of the other.
- Once upright move gently to where you wish to go, using a walking stick or an upright chair as a makeshift walking frame, if necessary.

Getting out of a chair

The process for getting out of a chair is similar — use your legs to straighten up and your hands in the small of your back to prevent you bending forward.

These manoeuvres are not easy, and for people in acute pain may prove almost impossible without help. However, if you can use them they will make life more comfortable, particularly once the back starts to heal.

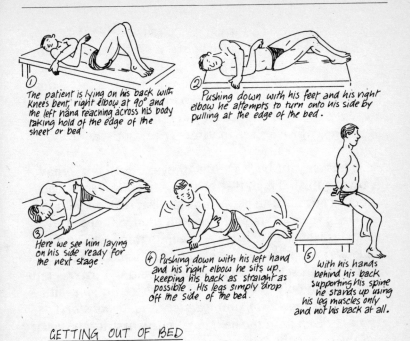

① The patient is lying on his back with knees bent, right elbow at 90° and the left hand reaching across his body taking hold of the edge of the sheet or bed.

② Pushing down with his feet and his right elbow he attempts to turn onto his side by pulling at the edge of the bed.

③ Here we see him laying on his side ready for the next stage.

④ Pushing down with his left hand and his right elbow he sits up. Keeping his back as straight as possible. His legs simply drop off the side of the bed.

⑤ With his hands behind his back supporting his spine he stands up using his leg muscles only and not his back at all.

GETTING OUT OF BED

Using the toilet

Using the toilet can sometimes be a problem during an acute attack. Men should sit down to pass water. Add bran and fibre to your diet to keep the stools as soft as possible to prevent straining on the toilet. This is important because the combination of pain, analgesics and bed rest causes the bowel to become sluggish.

If you can, get someone to put a low footstool or a couple of telephone directories in front of the toilet on which to rest your feet. Your body will then be in more of a squatting position, which should also make passing stools easier.

Sneezing and coughing

Sneezing and coughing can be agony when you are in acute pain. The best advice, apart from 'Don't!' is to look upwards so that you don't bend you head down as is usual when sneezing and coughing. It is also a good idea to grab hold of something solid, such as a chair, a table or the edge of the bed, so that you brace yourself for the shock.

Exercise

Lying in bed is both boring and bad for the muscles, which can get very stiff if they don't work. So many osteopaths suggest a gentle exercise routine to be practised for five minutes every hour.

Lie flat on your back with your eyes closed and breathe deeply, trying to let all the tension go from your muscles. Start by concentrating on your right leg, then on your right arm, then on your left leg, and then your left arm until your whole body is loose. Keep in mind what a rag doll looks like — that is the effect you should aim for. Now tighten the muscles of each foot and hand in turn, keeping them taut for only a few seconds before letting go again. *If your pain increases stop immediately and do not start the exercises again until the next day.* In the first few hours or so of the acute phase, any attempt at contracting muscle can be very painful indeed. However, if you are free of pain, continue by lying on your back pulling the toes of each foot in turn up towards you and holding the position for a count of five before relaxing again. Now push each arm into the bed in turn for a count of five seconds. Finish by slowly contracting and relaxing the buttock muscles twenty times.

BEFORE AND AFTER AN ACUTE ATTACK

Beds

We spend almost one third of our lives in bed and so it is very important to get the choice of bed right. Orthopaedic beds, some costing many hundreds of pounds, are made by most bed manufacturers, but most of them are extremely hard, which does not suit everyone.

When choosing a bed go to the largest bed shop or department store you can find. Lie down on all sorts of different beds and choose the one that suits you best. If you prefer a firm bed while your partner likes a softer one, there are several ranges that combine two different single beds that zip together. The best beds are divans with drawers underneath or slatted wooden beds, because the base is solid wood and the support therefore excellent. Any firm mattress (not an orthopaedic one) can be put on top and that is all you need. The mattress should be turned from side to side and from end to end each month if it is to last. And do remember that the life of a mattress is no more than eight years or so.

Hotel beds can be notoriously bad and this can be a problem if you do much travelling. If your hotel bed is too soft, ask the manager for a board to go under the mattress. Failing that put the mattress on the floor and sleep that way. It is better than having your back wreck your plans.

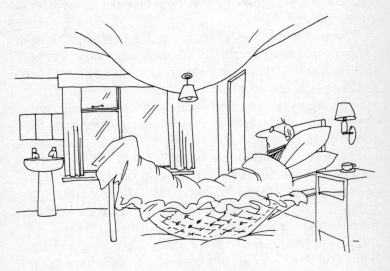

Hotel beds can be notoriously bad.

Putting pillows under your waist, or between your knees if you lie on your side, to keep your spine straight can also be quite helpful. Once again, experiment to find out what's best for you.

Pillows

Just as there are beds for back sufferers, so there are special neck pillows designed to help sufferers from arthritis or fibrositis. But again, they are not really much use. Instead, try sleeping on your side and bunching your pillow up so that your neck is well supported and level with your shoulders. In this way the muscles on both sides can relax and the joints are not stretched. Obviously pillows stuffed with feathers or foam chips are best for this, and the solid foam pillows unsuitable.

Problems around the house

Housework can be quite a problem for patients who suffer from chronic and acute back pain. If you're apt to be obsessive about housework, reduce the amount you do, although admittedly some things still have to be done! The following suggestions may help to make household chores easier.

Vacuuming involves a bending and a pushing action. Short people need an upright cleaner, while taller people need a cylindrical cleaner with an extra piece of rigid hose that helps them avoid bending. The use of a light carpet sweeper every day and the vacuum cleaner perhaps only once a week will reduce the amount of time you have to spend on this chore.

In the kitchen, use a step stool to reach things from high cupboards. Sit at a table to avoid standing while preparing food. If your kitchen doesn't have a table, try sitting at a work surface with your feet in a cupboard. Low ovens are a source of danger for the unwary. Many a Christmas has been ruined by lifting a heavy turkey from a low oven. Don't — get someone else to do it for you.

Laundry and washing can be very heavy when wet. Loading and unloading the washing machine involves bending and lifting, so again do get help if in doubt. Or else you can try squatting on your haunches, which will reduce the bending.

If you find that ironing gives you backache sitting down might help, but some people find this very difficult to do

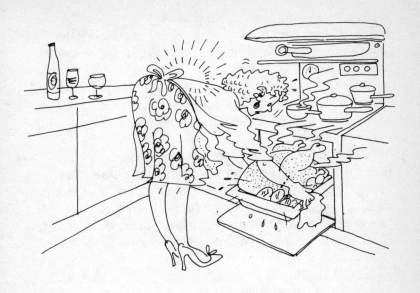

Low ovens are a source of danger...

and prefer to stand. Use a small box or a couple of telephone directories to rest your foot on. This means that you can take your weight on alternate sides, which may help. Also, ask yourself if all the things you are about to iron really need it.

Bed making is much easier if you use a duvet or a continental quilt, as you don't have to bend. If you haven't got duvets, make the bed kneeling down — though this is far from ideal.

Problems particular to women

If you are intending to do any heavy or strenuous activity, first consult your diary. Some 70 per cent of women and girls who experience an acute attack of low back pain for the first time do so within three days of a menstrual period. At this time the levels of the hormone progesterone are suddenly reduced so that the period can start, but one side effect of this completely normal process is a slight weakening effect of the ligaments of the pelvis and low back. So if possible try to avoid heavy work, particularly lifting at this time. If that is impossible remember that your back is not as strong as it normally is and be extra careful.

You may be among the small number of women who find that tampons aggravate a pre-existing low back problem. If this is the case, it may be better to use sanitary towels.

Occasionally low back pain associated with menstruation is caused by a gynaecological problem rather than a mechanical one. The details of your medical case history should enable the properly trained osteopath to assess your problem correctly (see page 50). However, if there is any doubt you will be referred back to your GP.

Sex and back pain

One possible cause of back pain that most people overlook is sex. Low back pain can be made much worse during sexual intercourse if either partner has a pre-existing low back problem and is not too careful.

In general, the partner who has no back pain should be the more active. The partner underneath should support the lumbar region of his or her spine with a cushion or pillow. The man should try not to thrust too deep as the rocking movements of his hips can strain his back. The woman should avoid pulling her knees up too far as this can flex the lumbar spine and cause a strain. If the woman is on top she should take her weight on her arms and not lean back too far as this can also cause strain. If the man is on top and his partner has a problem, he should take his weight on his arms or elbows to avoid hurting her. He should also take care to be gentle, as if he is too vigorous he can push his partner's pelvis and jar her spine.

If couples prefer a rear entry position, the woman should be supported by pillows to avoid straining her back, if she is the one with the problem. Again, take care not to jar her spine. Sometimes it is best if each partner lies on their side, as in this position neither has to take the full weight of the other.

Once again the best advice is to experiment to find out what is best for you both. And take comfort from the fact that most episodes of back pain do not last for very long.

Coping with a new baby

Many women find they start having back problems soon after they have their first baby. Coping with a new baby can be very strenuous as it involves lifting and bending at the wrong height and at the wrong angles, so it is not surprising that people hurt themselves.

Coping with a new baby is not just the mother's problem. Fathers become involved with nappy changing and feeding, so the following tips apply to men and women alike.

Change the baby's nappies as near as possible to chest height to avoid bending. It is possible to buy special changing tables, but they are expensive. It is probably best to change the baby on the bed while you are kneeling down. For cleanliness and hygiene the baby should be on a changing mat. Changing nappies in this way gives the baby room to roll over safely and prevents the parent having to bend from the waist.

Putting the baby into and taking it out of a cot can be difficult as most cots are low. Buy a cot with sides that drop, and then put the baby down in it while you are kneeling. Do the same when you want to pick the baby up again. Very young babies are quite safe in a drawer or carrycot on the dressing table, if it is firm enough, in the parents' bedroom. This, too, avoids unnecessary bending and lifting.

Baby baths are also too low. Why not take the baby into the bath with you or bath the baby in the sink in the kitchen? In both cases take care that the baby's head does not knock against the taps or sides of the bath or sink.

Baby slings that strap in front of the adult are not very good as they tend to pull the weight of the adult forward, so making the back muscles work harder to remain upright and causing them to ache more. It is far better to carry your baby on your back red-indian style.

Once your child has become a toddler, it is best to pick him or her up by getting down on your knees. Get your child to hug you as close as possible, then with one hand around the child and the other holding onto the cot or a chair stand up while trying to keep your back as straight as possible as you push yourself up using your leg muscles.

Feeding the baby is best done with your back well supported by pillows in a chair or on the bed. Do *not* lean over the child. It is common to see pictures of nursing mothers with their heads bent forward, straining their necks. It is not just low back strains that occur at this time — neck muscles are equally vulnerable.

The car

Long car journeys can be a nightmare for back sufferers and are always worse for the passengers. Drivers at least use their arm and leg muscles while driving, whereas passengers are stuck in one position for a long time.

If at all possible try to choose a car with good seats. The best car seats have adjustable back supports or at least an adjustment that alters the rake or angle of the whole seat back. Practically everyone when they get into a car, starts by sitting upright and supported, but after 20 minutes or so begins to slump down, leaving the lumbar spine unsupported. This is what leads to backache. Having the seat upright and, if you are driving, as close to the steering wheel as is safe, will help to correct this.

Allow sufficient time on the journey, so that every hour you can stop to stretch your legs and spine for two minutes. This will mean that you arrive at your destination free from backpain.

If you have a puncture, try to get help. Changing a wheel is a heavy, awkward task and should be undertaken very carefully by anyone with a back problem.

Cleaning and polishing the car involves a lot of effort. Don't do it until the acute phase of backpain is well out of

Could we use the car-jack to get you back in the car?

CHANGING A WHEEL IS A TASK TO BE UNDERTAKEN
VERY CAREFULLY BY ANYONE WITH A BACK PROBLEM.

the way. After all, your local car wash is cheaper than an osteopath's fees.

If you must do work on the car, make sure you have the correct tools for the job. Hire some if necessary, don't hope to get by as you generally do. Use a spray to loosen tight nuts and bolts, and using a longer lever than usual will mean less strain on your back. If the part you are changing is heavy, be sure to get some help in lifting it. And give yourself frequent breaks — leaning into the engine compartment without a break for longer then a quarter of an hour or so is asking for trouble.

DIY and decorating
Painting and decorating in themselves are harmless enough occupations but painting ceilings can be treacherous, particularly for people with neck problems. Avoid bending your neck as much as possible by using steps, scaffolding towers and trestles. Even a long handle on the end of your paint roller is better than bending your neck back.

Heavy DIY work, such as removing a wall to make a through lounge or removing chimneybreasts, really does need at least two people, both of whom should have reasonably fit backs.

Lastly, self-assembly furniture that comes in flat packs can be very heavy indeed and needs at least two people to lift and put it together.

Gardening

Gardening, although generally a healthy pastime, is not without its pitfalls. Always use long-handled tools when hoeing or digging, and if the ground is very hard leave the digging for another day. Prolonged bending, weeding or lifting vegetables, will almost certainly give you a backache. Instead, plan the jobs to be done and then alternate between, say, 20 minutes bending and 20 minutes in the greenhouse or potting shed. This will mean that you can work all morning or afternoon without facing an agonizing evening.

When using a rake or a broom, be careful not to be too vigorous with twisting and bending strokes. Even clearing up leaves can cause problems if not done carefully.

Approach all heavy lifting with caution — that sack of wet grass cuttings is heavier than you think.

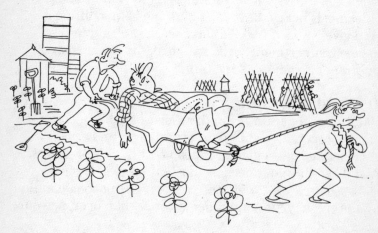

Gardening, although a really pleasant pastime, is not without its pitfalls ...

Baths

A good soak in a hot bath eases muscles after a hard bout of gardening or DIY. But when you get out of the bath after a long soak, don't dry yourself straight away. Your muscles will be very relaxed and as you twist and bend to dry yourself you could easily strain them. Instead, wrap up in a towel or bath sheet and put on your dressing gown. Lie down on the bed for half an hour and dry off in this way and then get dressed. You will not catch a cold if the room is warm and you'll feel much more relaxed.

Sport

Sport by definition encourages fitness. But some sports are decidedly dangerous for back pain sufferers. The table on page 86 shows sports grouped into three categories according to the risks involved and the demands they put on the back or the neck.

It is unwise for anyone with a history of back or neck problems to take part in any contact sport. In contrast, swimming is one of the best possible sports because it provides exercise while the water carries the body's

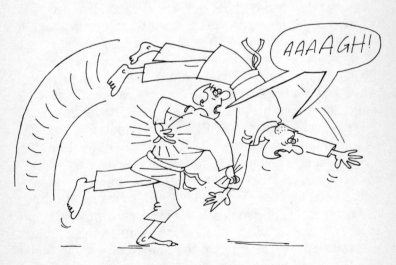

AAAAGH!

The martial arts – high risk for
back pain sufferers...

weight. Jogging is fine on grass, but marathon running is simply too much for chronic back pain sufferers. Surprisingly, snooker is not without risks because of the prolonged bending involved.

HIGH RISK	MEDIUM RISK	LOW RISK
Martial arts	Golf	Swimming
Boxing	Squash	Jogging
Rugby	Soccer	Tennis
Motor sport	Cricket	Cycling
Gymnastics	Ten-pin bowling	Bowls
Parachuting	Fencing	Table tennis
Hang gliding	Water polo	Badminton
Marathon running	Basketball	
Diving	Weight training	
Weight lifting	Aerobics	

Sports and their level of risk to back pain sufferers

Always do a series of back exercises as a warm up before going out, and do the same set when you get back to the changing room to warm down again afterwards. If you get muscular aches and pains the day after a heavy game, it is usually because you did not warm down after the game, and not because you have injured a muscle. If in doubt about suitable exercises, ask your osteopath.

If you feel a twinge, STOP! Do not think that you can run off an injury, you cannot. Professional players don't try to do this. They have professional trainers and advisers who treat them as soon as they leave the pitch. You do not, and the professionals were much fitter than you to start with. So remember, *pain is a warning sign and should never be ignored.* It is fairer to your team to declare yourself unfit before a match than have them try to find a substitute half way through.

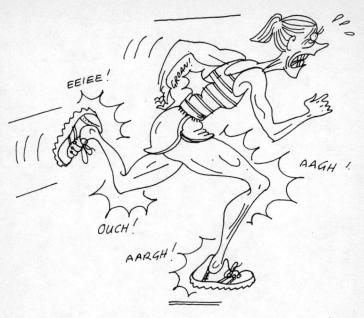

Pain is a warning sign and shouldn't be ignored.

Obesity and back pain

The spine and the discs have a number of functions to perform. The most important is the transmission of body weight to the legs and pelvis. It is therefore important that back sufferers should be very careful about their weight. There are no miraculous ways to lose weight, despite the number of books and magazines dealing solely with this subject. Your doctor or osteopath will advise you on the ideal weight for your age and frame. Be prepared to be patient — it may take a long time to lose the weight, but will be worth it!

7.
OSTEOPATHY AND THE MEDICAL WORLD

Sadly many people, medical and lay people alike, view alternative or complementary medicine of any sort, including osteopathy, with suspicion. This suspicion is born out of confusion of the facts regarding the scientific background to present day osteopathic research, and ignorance regarding the legality of referral from practitioners of orthodox medicine to practitioners of complementary therapy.

Research studies into each of the complementary medicines has failed because researchers have tried to approach research into complementary medicine with the same criteria as used in orthodox medicine.

It is all very well for orthodox medicine to use the system of double blind trials in which one group of patients takes the active drug while the other takes the placebo or blank drug, but how can you give a patient a blank osteopathic treatment?

Research into validating osteopathic treatment is currently being done at many of the hospitals attached to the major centres of osteopathic medicine in the USA and the results that have been obtained so far have gone a long way to giving scientific credence to the osteopathic principles that have been used by practitioners over the years.

As regards the legality of orthodox doctors referring patients to practitioners of complementary medicine, the situation was clarified by the GMC (General Medical Council) in January 1975. From that date doctors were given the authority to refer patients to whoever they wished, providing they recognized the fact that the individual was competent to practise in their field and that the doctor retained control of the case.

Here then is the real heart of the problem. Doctors and lay people often do not know how to distinguish the properly trained therapist from the others. The public are quite unprotected in this matter, because in Britain anyone who wants to set up as an osteopath, homeopath, acupuncturist or hypnotherapist, for example, can do so with impunity and no training whatsoever.

In 1936, on the advice of a House of Lords enquiry, the osteopathic profession was advised to set up its own register to safeguard the public and help remedy the situation. The Register, as it is known, represents the majority of full-time trained osteopaths practising in Britain today. In order to use the title 'Registered Osteopath' (a title protected under the law), it is necessary to have qualified from an approved school of training recognized and inspected by the GCRO (General Council and Register of Osteopaths).

Prospective patients will find the names and addresses of the recognized schools on page 99.

In the last few years osteopaths have been able, with the permission of patients and their GPs, to obtain X-rays and blood tests from hospitals. If it is not the hospital's policy to release this information, the osteopath can go to the hospital and study their files. It is still not possible for the osteopath to send the patient direct to the hospital for tests, as osteopathic treatment is still not available on the National Health Service.

Doctors are certainly beginning to appreciate that osteopathy is not a threat to their profession and may benefit their patients. Only ten years ago it was rare for an osteopath to have patients referred by a doctor, but now as many as half of all patients in some osteopathic practices come in this way. Now, too, some of the major private medical insurance groups recognize certain osteopaths and their fees are accepted for payment.

ALTERNATIVE MEDICINE OR COMPLEMENTARY MEDICINE?

Part of the reason why historically there has been conflict between osteopaths and doctors may lie in the unfortunate use of the term 'alternative medicine' to describe osteopathy. It suggests a division which should not exist. If you offer something as an alternative, it suggests a choice between one system and another. This need not be the case. Most osteopaths prefer the use of the phrase 'complementary medicine', which suggests a discipline running parallel to the existing system and neither replacing nor competing with it. Complementary medicine adds to the existing system without taking anything away.

An excellent example of this can be found in the work some osteopaths do with pregnant women. Back pain is a very common complaint in pregnancy and drugs or corsets, which are the standard medical treatments for the non-pregnant back pain sufferer, are out of the question. Likewise bedrest for prolonged periods is often not possible either. Osteopaths have found, however, that gentle manipulation of the pelvic and spinal joints, together with the soft tissue techniques described on page 61, can dramatically reduce the pain caused by carrying the extra weight on the loose ligaments of the pelvis and spine. The patient will also be given advice and treatment aimed at restoring good postural tone, to

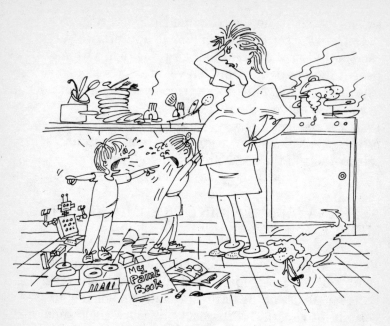

Osteopathy can often help pregnant women suffering from back pain when bed-rest is probably not possible.

prevent the condition recurring.

As far as the future is concerned, before too long there will be legislation recognizing the osteopathic profession as an independent body. There will soon be osteopaths working in NHS hospitals and health centres, alongside GPs — paid for by the NHS and not the patient. The only restraint to this now is financial, but with pressure from patients who demand this sort of care, it will soon become a reality.

OSTEOPATHY AND PHYSIOTHERAPY

People often confuse the work of osteopaths and physiotherapists. The two professions do have many similarities, but there are also important differences. For example, a physiotherapist is not trained to make a diagnosis, only an assessment of the patient's condition.

That is why, traditionally, a patient never went directly to a physiotherapist, but was always first referred by a doctor. Osteopaths, however, treat as practitioners in their own right and have been trained to make their own diagnoses and assessments as a matter of course. They make their own decisions about whom to treat and whom to refer on and in this respect osteopaths carry a greater degree of responsibility for their patients than do physiotherapists.

Physiotherapists use many other methods of treatment apart from their hands. They use heat, cold, machines to massage muscles, traction apparatus, ultrasound and short-wave diathermy, as well as exercises after treatment. Some osteopaths also use electrical apparatus, but not to the same extent as physiotherapists do.

Physiotherapists work in every department of a hospital and one of their most important jobs is helping with post-operative recovery and recuperation — making sure that the patient is breathing well and helping to prevent infection setting in. They work in rehabilitation departments helping patients recover from accidents or relearning how to walk after limb surgery or the fitting of an artificial limb.

Osteopathy and physiotherapy are no threat to each other. Each profession has a different role to serve. Osteopaths are trained in independent diagnosis, looking much more for the cause of the problem. Their priorities are very different from those of physiotherapists, when it comes to looking for the reasons why patients become ill or are in pain. Some patients, for example those with sports injuries that need weight training to build up torn or damaged muscles, would respond better to physiotherapy than to osteopathic treatment.

Many osteopaths have very good relationships with physiotherapists working in their area — relationships based on mutual trust and respect for each other's role. This is best for the patient, the two professions and for medicine in general.

8.
HOW TO FIND A PRACTITIONER

The information given in this chapter will help you to find a reliable, qualified osteopath. Please note that organizations offering lists of practitioners usually request a stamped addressed envelope.

THE REGISTER OF OSTEOPATHS

The General Council and Register of Osteopaths (GCRO) was founded in 1936. It is the osteopathic profession's governing body — regulating educational standards, exercising ethical control over its members and protecting the public from charlatanism.

From its inception the Register has been concerned with the supervision of those training schools who wish their graduating students to be able to practise as members of the Register of Osteopaths and thus use the initials MRO after their name.

By keeping a directory of practitioners, it enables

members of the public to know that there is an acceptable standard that members of the Register aspire to, so the public can be assured of a level of safety and competence. This does not mean that those practitioners who are not MROs are necessarily charlatans. All it tells the public is that they do not have the standards laid down by the GCRO. There are other organizations that have their own ethical standards, but as they have not applied to the GCRO for inspection and thus inclusion within the Register, the GCRO cannot endorse their registers or their members.

The title 'Registered Osteopath' is protected in law and there have been successful court cases in the past where the GCRO has maintained the right of its members and its members alone to use these words on notepaper or appointment cards.

There is a convention in Britain that members of the medical professions do not advertise, a convention that also applies to Registered Osteopaths. There are, however, two exceptions. Newly qualified graduates setting up a practice, or established members who change their address are permitted to advertise, but the form of the advertisement is strictly controlled by the Register and members who contravene this code of ethics risk a fine or in serious cases suspension or expulsion.

Copies of the directory listing Registered Osteopaths can be found in most public libraries or Citizens Advice Bureaux. They can also be obtained from:

The Secretary
The General Council and Register of Osteopaths
21 Suffolk Street
London SW1
Tel: 01-839 2060

OSTEOPATHY TRAINING

The precise curriculum varies between the different osteopathy training schools, but all thorough courses, including those at schools recognized by the GCRO, cover the following topics:

The basic science course

This course covers human anatomy, applied histology, embryology, biochemistry and physiology. The students attend lecture demonstrations in the dissecting rooms of well-known teaching hospitals and practical classes are held at colleges of further education. The students also attend classes in osteopathic technique, where they learn the basic handling skills and elementary manipulation techniques of normal tissue. The students all practise these skills on each other. Any student who does not meet the minimum pass standard in all subjects at the regular examinations is required to leave the course at that stage.

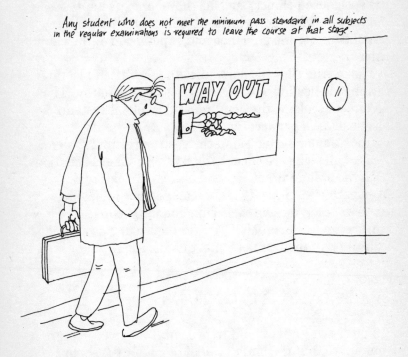

Any student who does not meet the minimum pass standard in all subjects in the regular examinations is required to leave the course at that stage.

The pre-clinical course

This course is designed to prepare the students for their work in the school's outpatient clinic. They start to look at the pathological changes that take place in the human body suffering from diseases, and the diagnostic points to lead them to an accurate assessment of the patient before treatment. They learn how to use blood tests and X-rays, the use of the stethoscope and opthalmoscope and how to examine each of the body's systems. Lectures and tutorials are given in the principles of osteopathy and in osteopathic diagnosis. Tuition in osteopathic technique continues, as the students begin to learn more complicated treatment techniques.

The clinical course
This is the longest part of most courses. Students spend more than 1500 hours working in their training school's busy outpatient clinics, both in the general clinic and in the specialized clinics, such as those for expectant mothers and for sports injuries. Senior students treat patients under the guidance and supervision of the clinic tutors.

During the clinical course the students attend lectures in subjects dealing with the practice of osteopathy. These include pathology, the neuromusculoskeletal system, obstetrics and gynaecology, respiratory and cardiovascular systems and the gastrointestinal system.

Students who are successful in their final examinations, both theory and practical, and can satisfy external osteopathic examiners of their competence in dealing with patients, then receive their Diploma in Osteopathy. They can then put the initials DO after their name as an indication of their professional qualification.

QUALIFICATIONS IN OSTEOPATHY

When seeking advice and treatment from an osteopath, do make sure that the initials appearing after the osteopath's name appear in the list opposite.

DO   — Diploma in Osteopathy
MRO   — Member of the Register of Osteopaths
MLCOM   — Member of the London College of
              Osteopathic Medicine
MBNOA   — Member of the British Naturopathic and
              Osteopathic Association
BSO   — British School of Osteopathy
ESO   — European School of Osteopathy
BCNO   — British College of Osteopathy and
              Naturopathy

USEFUL ADDRESSES

Information and advice
The General Council and Register of Osteopaths
21 Suffolk Street
London SW1
Tel: 01-839 2060

The British Naturopathic and Osteopathic Association
Frazer House
6 Netherhall Gardens
London NW3
Tel: 01-435 7830

Clinics with full-time recognized training
The British School of Osteopathy
Littlejohn House
1-4 Suffolk Street
London SW1
Tel: 01-930 9254

The European School of Osteopathy
104 Tonbridge Road
Maidstone
Kent
Tel: (0622) 671558

The Osteopathic Association Clinic
8 Boston Place
London NW1
Tel: 01-262 1128

Osteopathy is practised in several countries around the world. Many of these countries have their own associations and registers. Information about osteopathy and local practitioners can be obtained from:

CANADA

Canadian Osteopathic Association
575 Waterloo Street
London
Ontario
N6 B2 R2

AUSTRALIA

Australian Osteopathic Association
551 Hampton Street
Hampton
Victoria 3188

This is the address of one of the main organizations representing osteopathy in Australia. However, each state still retains its right to recognize its own members. Someone who is qualified to practise in Sydney might not be qualified to practise in Melbourne. There are also a number of practising osteopaths, who have trained and registered in the UK. They will have the initials MRO after their names.

NEW ZEALAND

Register of New Zealand Osteopaths
c/o Robert Bowden
92 Hurtsmere Road
Takapuna
Auckland

Osteopaths registered with this organization use the initials MNZRO after their names. There are also some English trained practitioners who can be recognized by the initials MRO after their names.

INDEX

ABOUT THE AUTHOR

STEPHEN SANDLER, DO, MRO, is a registered osteopath in private practice. He is also Head of the Expectant Mothers' Unit and Head of the Department of Osteopathic Practice at the British School of Osteopathy in London.

He has written several research papers on aspects of osteopathy. This is his first book.

He lives in north London, with his wife and two children.

More books from Optima

FRIENDS OF THE EARTH HANDBOOK
edited by Jonathon Porritt
A great many people are interested in protecting the
environment, but are not sure what they should do about it.
This is a practical guide on how to put environmental ideals into
practice.
  Topics discussed include the best ways to save energy, waste
disposal, the use of water, transport policies, the protection of
wildlife and the politics of food.
ISBN 0 356 12560 2
Price (in UK only) **£4.95**

THE HOSPICE WAY by Denise Winn
Public interest in hospices and the care of the terminally ill is
growing.
  Denise Winn explains in a sympathetic way what hospice
care means, the aims and philosophy of hospices, and how these
are put into effect, including the control of pain, the underlying
acceptance of death, and the welcome extended to patients'
families and friends.
  Advice is given on how to find a hospice, and at what stage,
any financial arrangements, and the possibility of hospice-style
care at home.
ISBN 0 356 12741 9
Price (in UK only) **£3.95**

YOUR BRILLIANT CAREER by Audrey Slaughter
This handbook by Audrey Slaughter, well-known Fleet Street
editor, offers a wealth of very practical advice for women of all
ages on how to turn a job into a career, with information about
training and specific management skills, as well as self-
confidence and mental attitude.
  The book includes useful hints from women at the top, and
will be of real help to all working women.
ISBN 0 356 12705 2
Price (in UK only) **£4.95**

STONE AGE DIET by Leon Chaitow
Leon Chaitow, well-known nutritionist and author, explores the
idea that the diet of our Stone Age ancestors was not only
healthy, enabling them to develop the most stable society known

in world history, but also very much in keeping with modern nutritional advice.

The book is firmly based on the latest scientific research, and includes a number of appropriate recipes.
ISBN 0 356 12328 6
Price (in UK only) **£4.95**

SELF HELP WITH PMS by Dr Michelle Harrison
One of the most comprehensive books available on the subject of PMS (premenstrual syndrome), it covers *all* its symptoms, both physical and mental, including the much publicized topic of premenstrual tension. The forms of treatment are fully described in clear, everyday language. Case histories and up-to-date details of new research into treatment are also included.

Illustrated with humorous but sympathetic line drawings, this book is an indispensable guide for the large number of women who suffer from this syndrome every month.
ISBN 0 356 12559 9
Price (in UK only) **£5.95**

MENOPAUSE THE NATURAL WAY by Dr Sadja Greenwood
A comprehensive book that answers all the questions a woman could possibly ask about the menopause. Myths about the menopause are corrected and all medical details are clearly explained in language that anyone can understand. All forms of treatment for the problems associated with the menopause are discussed, including the most up-to-date and controversial. Includes case histories and is illustrated with humorous but sympathetic line drawings, that complement the positive approach of the book.

It will be welcomed by every woman (and a lot of men) as a complete, practical guide to promoting good health and avoiding illness in the second half of life.
ISBN 0 356 12561 0
Price (in UK only) **£5.95**

ALTERNATIVE HEALTH SERIES
This series is designed to provide factual information and practical advice about alternative therapies. While including essential details of theory and history, the books concentrate on what patients can expect during treatment, how they should prepare for it, what questions will be asked and why, what form

the treatment will take, what it will 'feel' like and how soon they can expect to respond.

1. ACUPUNCTURE by Michael Nightingale
Acupuncture is a traditional Chinese therapy which usually (but not always) uses needles to stimulate the body's own energy and so bring healing.
ISBN 0 356 12426 6
Price (in UK only) **£3.95**

   This book, OSTEOPATHY by Stephen Sandler, is also part of the series.

BELOW THE BELT — A WOMAN'S GUIDE TO GENITO-URINARY INFECTIONS by Denise Winn
A simple factual guide to all the sexually transmitted diseases and vaginal infections women risk catching.
   It covers all the long recognized diseases, such as gonorrhoea and syphilis, and the most up-to-date facts about all the new hazards — herpes, genital warts, chlamydia and AIDS.
   Causes, symptoms in both yourself and your partner, and advice on treatment (including self-help) are clearly explained, as are the possible consequences of not seeking treatment.
   A frank and direct account, firmly based on the latest medical knowledge.
ISBN 0 356 12740 0
Price (in UK only) **£3.95**

DOWN TO EARTH — A CALENDAR FOR THE RELUCTANT GARDENER by Mike Gilliam with Alan Titchmarsh
DOWN TO EARTH, like the associated radio programme, is for every gardener who only wants to potter for a couple of hours at the weekend, and still expects results. There's one main, illustrated job for each week, plus topical tips on smaller 'odd jobs'. The style is lively, the approach not always orthodox, and subjects range widely — lawns, hedges, flowers, ponds, trees, even discouraging unwelcome cats. The emphasis is on the easy, instant results and maximum effect for minimum cost and effort.
ISBN 0 356 12704 4
Price (in UK only) **£4.95**

All Optima books are available at your bookshop or newsagent, or can be ordered from the following address:

Optima, Cash Sales Department,
P.O. Box 11, Falmouth, Cornwall.

Please send cheque or postal order (no currency), and allow 55p for postage and packing for the first book plus 22p for the second book and 14p for each additional book ordered up to a maximum charge of £1.75 in U.K.

Customers in Eire and B.F.P.O. please allow 55p for the first book, 22p for the second book plus 14p per copy for the next 7 books, thereafter 8p per book.

Overseas customers please allow £1 for postage and packing for the first book and 25p per copy for each additional book.